MANUAL THERAPY

"NAGS", "SNAGS",

"MWMS" etc.

Brian R Mulligan
FNZSP (Hon), Dip MT

Third Edition

First published 1989
Revised 2nd Edition 1992
Revised 3rd Edition 1995

© Plane View Services Ltd., 22 Westview Grove, Wellington, New Zealand

ISBN 0-473-03039-X

Printing and typesetting: Hutcheson Bowman & Stewart Ltd

To my wife Dawn
who encouraged me
to rewrite this book.

THE AUTHOR

Brian R Mulligan qualified as a registered physiotherapist in 1954 and gained his Diploma in Manipulative Therapy in 1974. In 1996 he was made an Honorary Fellow of The New Zealand Society of Physiotherapists for his contribution to physiotherapy.

He together with R A McKenzie and J C Cameron established The New Zealand Manipulative Therapists' Association in 1968 and was made a life member of this body in 1988.

Apart from his private practice in Wellington he has been involved in the teaching of manual therapy in New Zealand since 1970. He has been teaching manual therapy internationally since 1972 and his courses have always proved popular. To meet the huge demand from therapists wishing to learn his techniques and to ensure high standards he set up an international organisation in 1995 to accredit teachers. Participants on courses conducted by those accredited would be assured of a high teaching standard.

Brian Mulligan has been the author of numerous articles that have appeared in issues of The New Zealand Journal of Physiotherapy and overseas publications. His first video titled "Manual Therapy" was produced in 1990 and his second "Mobilisations with Movement" in 1993.

In 1996 he was made an Honorary Fellow of The New Zealand Society of Physiotherapists for his contribution to physiotherapy.

CONTENTS

PART TWO

THE EXTREMITIES. MOBILISATIONS WITH MOVEMENT. (MWMs)

PART THREE

THE EXTREMITIES. A POT POURRI

A. COMPESSION TREATMENTS FOR EXTREMITY JOINTS

B. PAIN RELEASE PHENOMENON TECHNIQUES - "PRP"s

PREFACE

Yet again I have put pen to paper to bring out another (third) edition of my book on manual therapy.

This has been done for two reasons. The first is to acquaint all therapists, practicing in the musculo-skeletal field, of technique improvements as well as my latest procedures. Secondly I wish to more than emphasize the importance of this whole new field of 'Mobilisation with Movements' (MWMs). It began of course with "SNAGS" which was a spinal mobilisation with spinal movement. I then found that MWMs had a exciting place in the treatment of extremities. The reader will now find that MWMs for virtually all the joints in the body are covered in this book . For those of you who treat the spine the latest MWM approaches, where mobilisations of the spine are combined with upper or lower limb movements, are often the safest and best manual therapy techniques you can use. Indications for them are carefully detailed .

Another point I must stress in this edition is that, with the exception of PRP'S, all the techniques in the book are painless. This is quite different from the often quoted phrase "No gain no pain".

In updating this manual I am again assuming that the reader . . .

1. Is fully aware of the contraindications to manual therapy and abides by the rules.

2 Has a sound knowledge of anatomy and biomechanics.

3. Has confident handling and language skills as without them the patient will not relax or comply with instructions. Poor handling can negate the advantages of manual therapy.

It is stating the obvious to say that many different manual therapy concepts and procedures are taught and in writing my book I was very conscious of this. However all the techniques in this publication are expected, when indicated and used, to bring about an immediate improvement in the patient's condition. A failure to do so would suggest the techniques are not appropriate for this patient or perhaps have not been undertaken correctly. On all my courses I say to participants that if no improvement is evident at the time of delivery then discard the technique and try another approach and they should not be continued if some of the improvement gained was not retained between visits. Endless perseverance with no lasting benefits cannot be justified. Spectacular results are often attained when using MWMs and I expect in my practice at least one "miracle" a day using them.

In the preface to the 2nd edition I stated that my favourite technique was the "SQUEEZE" for the knee. Currently my 'sprained lateral ligament ' of the ankle findings take pride of place because we have discovered that about one in three patients presenting with this diagnosis have been misdiagnosed and the trauma is to the distal Tibio-fibular joint and the ligament itself is not involved. You must read on!

PART ONE

1. SPINAL MOBILISATIONS

Introduction

It is interesting to note that in the field of manual therapy, when spinal manipulations are taught, attention is paid to the movement planes of the facet joints.

The direction of one's thrust is related to these planes especially when rotation and side flexion techniques are used. When one considers the various mobilisations that are taught much less attention is paid to the facet planes. These comments are generalisations, I know, but they lead me to say that the mobilisations that I use are always applied at right angles or parallel to the treatment planes of the facet joints. This complies with rule that applies for extremity joint mobilisations as described in Freddy M Kaltenborn's book "Mobilisations of the Extremity Joints". (1) Here he describes the treatment plane as lying across the concave articular surface.

The treatment plane moves with the concave partner. It behoves physiotherapists to be familiar with the direction of all spinal facet planes. As you read further you will observe that all the spinal mobilisations are done with the patient weightbearing (In standing or sitting). I consider this to be extremely important as so often with non weightbearing techniques, improvements gained are lost when the patients resume an erect posture. Although not mentioned in this text other forms of appropriate physiotherapy would be given concurrently by the author. At this juncture I must point out that I do not use my mobilisations on two regularly encountered spinal conditions because there are more appropriate treatments available. These are the acute wry neck (acute torticollis) which I will deal with separately and the lumbar lesion producing a sciatic scoliosis (lateral shift) which is adequately dealt with using the R A McKenzie methods described in his book "The Lumbar Spine" (2).

A. THE CERVICAL AND UPPER THORACIC SPINES.

1. *"NAGS"*

Explanation

"NAGS" is the name I have given to oscillatory mobilisations which can be applied to the facet joints between Cervical 2 and Thoracic 3. It has become an acronym for "Natural Apophyseal Glides". Although no problem will be encountered in their execution in the cervical spine, therapists with short arms and small hands may not be able to use them in the upper thoracic spine.

"NAGS" are mid-range to end-range facet joint mobilisations that are applied antero-superiorly along the treatment planes of the joints selected. They are graded according to the tolerance of the patient. They must never cause pain, maybe minimal discomfort.

The patient is always seated which is a most convenient starting position. This is much more acceptable than prone lying especially with khyphotic patients. If discomfort is experienced traction can be applied with "NAGS" which really is a bonus. They are used to increase spinal movement and decrease the pain associated with it. They are very useful in the elderly when applied with tender loving care. For the patient with grossly restricted spinal movement they can prove a godsend, assuming that the loss of movement is not due to serious structural injury or other contraindicated pathology. In the middle-aged patient with end range movement pain, be it unilateral or bilateral , "NAGS" to the upper thoracic spine is usually the area of choice. The upper thoracic spine is often overlooked when dealing with neck restrictions. Soreness after a manipulative procedure will usually be relieved by "NAGS". They are often combined with "REVERSE NAGS" or in conjunction with "SNAGS" both of which will be described later.

Description (see figures 1a and 1b)

The patient is seated comfortably on a stool or chair. To accommodate different sizes of patients it would help if the seat was height adjustable.

You, the therapist, (if right handed) stand at the right side of the patient so that your lower trunk is in contact with the antero-lateral surface of the patient's right shoulder. This is to stabilise the trunk of the patient when the mobilisation is carried out.

The patient's head is cradled against your upper abdomen or chest, comfortably held there with the right forearm diagonally positioned across the left side of the patient's temporo-mandibular joint. As some contact is made with the therapist's lower chest the female operator would be wise to place a soft pad between her and a male patient's face for obvious reasons. I always place a paper tissue between my white coat and the patient's face not only for hygiene reasons but to capture the cosmetics worn by some. In positioning the head, rotation and side flexion should be avoided. The middle or terminal phalanx of your right little finger is now placed (hooked) just under the spinous process of the vertebra on top of the joint to be mobilised. (To mobilise the Cervical 5/6 joint your phalanx would be under the spinous process of Cervical 5) The right index and third fingers wrap around the occiput if your hand is large enough, to maximise firm contact with the patient's head.

The right arm also controls the degree of neck flexion. When more flexion is applied say to make better contact with a chosen spinous process, you must remember that you have altered the direction of the facet planes. The lateral border of the thenar eminence of your left hand is placed more under than over the little finger of your right hand. The required glide along the treatment plane can now be given, via your attached little finger, by pushing up and forward with your left hand. The wrist of your left arm should be in extension with the forearm sloping in the direction of the facet planes. The glides may be rhythmical (say three per second) or held for a few seconds at the end range of the movement.

When gliding rhythmically stay in the mid to end range of the movement.

Remember that the patient's trunk is stabilised with your body.

Care must be taken to ensure that the glides follow the true direction of the treatment plane as failure to do so will produce pain. If one thrusts ventrally first before gliding up correctly in a cranio-dorsal direction patients will feel unacceptable pain. I find this a common mistake made by therapists when I am teaching the technique.

The mobilisations are repeated 6-10 times and then joint movements are reassessed. Sometimes several sets are required to bring about a change.

As with all forms of manual therapy if no improvement is discernible then some other therapy would be given. Of course you may have chosen the wrong level and with some patients several levels may be involved.

If the patient experiences some discomfort with "NAGS" this can usually be eliminated by the addition of traction. This is done by cradling the patient's head to the body with your knees slightly flexed and then extending the knees or by slightly side flexing your trunk away from the patient.

This method of applying traction will be familiar to manual therapists.

The main advantage of this technique, apart from its efficacy, is its adaptability. Not only can it be applied with traction and various degrees of flexion or extension but one can introduce degrees of rotation or side flexion. The little finger may be placed over the articular pillar on one side to perform unilateral "NAGS" to restore side flexion or rotation.

For older patients in particular, with end range losses of rotation, unilateral "NAGS" to the upper thoracic spine are most rewarding. Cradle the head of the patient as before and place your fully flexed proximal inter phalangeal joint of your right little finger on the articular pillar on the restricted side. It should lie close to the spinous process at the suspected level. (see figure 1b) Place the thenar eminence of your free hand over the flexed 5th finger. Push firmly anteriorly to secure it to the articular pillar and then glide rhythmically up.

The right forearm fixating the head should be secure enough to enable some traction to be given if required.

"NAGS" have been described by my colleagues who have mastered them as extremely useful and I would try them on most of my patients with cervical and upper dorsal problems; particularly on those with a gross loss of movement or on the elderly. Only once in over twenty years has a patient of mine had an adverse reaction to "NAGS". When this occurred I used "REVERSE NAGS" (to be described in the next section) and the patient was better immediately. The reaction was really memorable. A 37 year old man presented with bilateral pain and a marked loss of movement in all directions. I applied gentle "NAGS" and the result was a further reduction in his range of movement. "REVERSE NAGS" were then used and his symptoms virtually disappeared. The reader would be interested to know that I again tried "NAGS" (gently of course) and his symptoms returned. "REVERSE NAGS" again relieved his symptoms. After his second visit two days latter no further therapy was required as he had fully recovered.

Figure 1a
"NAGS" to the mid cervical spine.

Figure 1b

Hand placement for unilateral "NAGS" to the upper thoracic spine.

2. "REVERSE NAGS"

Explanation

As the name implies these mobilisations are almost the reverse of "NAGS". If the latter prove unsuccessful then this technique should be tried. It is particularly useful in the cervical and upper thoracic spines in about 10% of patients on whom you would wish to try mobilisations.

Description. (See figures 2a and 2b)

The patient is seated. You stand beside the patient and cradle his head to your body with the forearm. Wrap your fifth finger around the posterior part of the vertebra above the suspected lesion. The free hand is clenched in such a way that a Vee is made between the thumb and flexed index finger. This Vee is placed over the spinous process of the vertebrae below the lesion.

This places the end of the thumb and the flexed index finger on the articular pillar each side. A mobilisation takes place when you glide the inferior facet up on the superior one. This is achieved by thrusting up along the treatment plane with your bottom hand. With "NAGS" the superior facet at the site of the lesion is moved up on the one below. With "REVERSE NAGS" the inferior facet moves up on the one above.

Figure 2a

"REVERSE NAGS" This illustrates the Vee between the thumb and index fingers.

Figure 2b

"REVERSE NAGS" to the mid cervical spine.

3. "SNAGS"

Explanation

"SNAGS" is an acronym for "Sustained Natural Apophyseal Glides". They are useful as a treatment for the cervical and upper thoracic spines. "SNAGS" for the lumbar and thoracic spines will be described later. Cervical "SNAGS" were a learning experience for me. They were the first example of what has become a new approach in the field of manual therapy and that is the combination of mobilisation with movement (MWM). What began as a unique technique for the cervical spine was found to have an important place in the treatment of other spinal joints. Because of their success there had to be a place for mobilisations with movement in the extremity joints and there certainly is. These will be dealt with under the extremity section of this book. "SNAGS" have yet to be scientifically vindicated but are never the less useful, safe, painless, easy to apply and a great introduction to this concept of mobilisation with movement. (The acronym has caught on. It is brief, explicit and when writing up case notes the only added description needed is to mention the level being treated. Thus my notes say "SNAGS" right rotation Cx 6/7. If "SNAGS" were unilaterally applied this would be recorded thus; "SNAGS" left rotation (r) Cx 6/7.) To assist in the promotion of "SNAGS" and other mobilisations with movement I am gathering a library of video evidence of their usefulness as they are applied to patients in my clinic. Although there are many texts available on spinal manual therapy I know of none which describe techniques that meet all the criteria that are listed below and thus the claim that "SNAGS" are a new approach. These are . . .

1. They are weightbearing.
2. They are mobilisations which are combined with active or passive movements and at the end of an active range overpressure is applied.
3. They follow the treatment plane rule that applies to extremity joints.
4. They are sustained.
5. They can be applied to most spinal joints.
6. When indicated they are PAINLESS. Any pain associated with the movement taking place is eliminated.
7. They are carried out at end range.
8. With a couple of movements you can decide if they are useful.
9. There is a straight forward procedure for each spinal movement loss.

This list must now be discussed in more detail for clarification.

1. They are weight bearing. All the texts that I have read on mobilisation have the patient lying. With "SNAGS" all procedures are done with the patient either sitting or standing. This has real advantages. When improvements take place in a functional posture they are more

likely to be retained. Before using "SNAGS" I found that while more conventional mobilisations can result in an immediate improvement in function while the patient is lying, it is often lost when they resume a weightbearing posture.

2. They are mobilisations with active or passive movement. At the end of the attainable active range of movement the patient would then assist by applying overpressure to further increase the movement. This overpressure enhances the response to the therapy.

3. They follow the treatment plane rule. This rule must be observed. Trying to glide facet joints outside this plane is incorrect. You will find that patients will be unable to move their necks actively without pain while applying an incorrect glide.

4. They are sustained. Most physiotherapy mobilisations for the spine are oscillatory. ie Maitland. "SNAGS" are mobilisations where the facet glides taking place are sustained while active and/or passive movement is taking place and these glides are maintained until the joint returns to the starting position. As an example, if Cervical 5/6 was being "SNAGGED" for a loss of extension then the therapist must sustain the glide with the movement until the neck resumes its resting position. Failure to do so might result in a painful response although no damage would occur. When a patient reaches end range active movement and compliments this with overpressure while you are gliding the facets, have him sustain this position for several seconds to further enhance the result.

5. They can be applied to most spinal joints. Yes they have a place in treating all the joints between the occiput and the sacrum.

6. When indicated they are painless. The indication for "SNAGS" is based on this statement which is in fact the rule governing their application. An explanation to the patient and his co-operation is essential for them to be successful. If there is any pain with a mobilisation with movement then STOP. You will never exacerbate a patient if you follow this rule. Remember of course that the pain may be produced because you have not followed the treatment plane rule or you may be mobilising the wrong segment.

7. They are carried out at end range. Mobilisations are usually undertaken with joints in a resting position. "SNAGS" are always involved with the end range of joint movement. If normal end range is lost it is expected when applying "SNAGS" that the movement loss will disappear or be dramatically reduced and that no pain will be felt. If the restriction does not alter then you would be wasting your time to proceed further. Try some other form of manual therapy. These techniques are so good that when indicated an improvement will be observed with the very first mobilisation with movement.

8. There is a straight forward procedure for each movement loss. When familiar with the techniques you will immediately know which one to apply when there is a painful movement loss.

9. Within a couple of minutes you can decide if "SNAGS" have a place in your treatment regime. If testing shows a painful loss of neck extension and right side flexion then "SNAGS" for these losses would be tried. Provided you are on the right level the pain with movement should go and the range increase straight away. If there is any pain check the level and technique. If still painful "SNAGS" would not be indicated. This routine takes only a short time.

Before continuing on might I again remind the reader that "SNAGS" like other manual therapies are only part of the treatment program for patients presenting with musculo-skeletal disorders.

Description

The best way to describe all "SNAGS" techniques is to relate them to their application and this is how they will be dealt with.

As with all therapies an explanation must be given to the patient before treatment is undertaken. The success of "SNAGS" and all other techniques dealt with in this book is totally dependant on the co-operation of the patient. To oblige they must be fully conversant with what you are doing and the most important feature to stress is that the technique of combining mobilisation with movement MUST BE PAINLESS. Pain of course may be experienced for many reasons and these must be checked out. As already mentioned you may have chosen the wrong level or the direction of your glide may be incorrect. Another point is that your handling rather than the technique may be at fault. If tissues are tender to the touch of your fingers or hands a thin layer of plastic foam may be placed under them. Finally "SNAGS" are not a cure all for all spinal mechanical disorders and should never be used if they produce pain.

(1) To increase rotation and/or decrease the pain associated with it. (See figure 3)

The patient is seated and you stand behind him. The medial border of one thumb's distal phalanx is placed on the tip of the spinous process of the vertebra above the suspected site of the lesion. Your other thumb reinforces this. This means that if the patient has a lesion at Cervical 5/6 your thumb would be on the Cervical 5's spinous process. The border of your thumb is used because the spinous processes are very small and the pulpy terminal pad would not be selective enough as it is too wide. Your other fingers are comfortably placed laterally on each side of the neck or upper antero-lateral thorax. You now glide the spinous process up in the direction of the treatment plane. The energy for this comes from the superimposed thumb pushing up on its partner. While this glide is being maintained ask the patient to turn his head in the restricted painful direction. As the head rotates you must follow with your hands to ensure that the mobilisation with the movement taking place remains along the treatment plane. Insist that the patient turns his neck slowly to enable you to maintain your glide up along the treatment plane. If "SNAGS" are indicated and the technique is correct the patient will be able to rotate his head further and feel no pain. Sustain, for several seconds, this new pain free end range of rotation, before returning to the midline. Repeat several times and then reassess. Unassisted active movement should now be much better.

"SNAGS" really are exciting when indicated. However do not overmobilise. Once an improvement has been obtained on the patient's first visit, stop. As with other forms of manual therapy they are often sore the next day. However if this is the case the discomfort is of short duration and I would repeat the therapy two days later. Patients may complain of local tenderness under your thumb but if the right joint is being "SNAGGED" that is all that they will feel. It is rare for this technique not to assist but as with all forms of manual therapy if no change is apparent at the time of delivery then it should be abandoned. "SNAGS" are diagnostically helpful in inculpating the level(s) of involvement as pressure applied to the wrong level will make no difference. It is amazing that a weight bearing combination of active movement with mobilisation can be so demonstratively effective.

Figure 3

"SNAGS" for cervical rotation.

Variations

Since the first edition of this book was published we have found a very satisfactory way for patients to effectively "SELF SNAG" their cervical spines and this will be described later in this section. When "SNAGS" are applied through the spinous process they are of course a bilateral technique. This is because both facets are equally glided. They can be effectively applied to the articular pillar on a chosen side. You still use your thumbs as you did over the spinous process. It would seem more logical to apply them unilaterally as spinal lesions usually only involve one side. In the case of a patient with painful right rotation you would initially unilaterally "SNAG" on the right side. If this did not work then try the pillar on the left. If again you have no success then "SNAG" through the spinous process, as already stated. To increase the efficacy of "SNAGS" for rotation, have the patient apply overpressure by using one of his hands to push the head further round and sustain this position for several seconds... After say six "SNAGS" with overpressure there should be a marked improvement in neck function and if not dispense with them.

At this point in the text I would like to mention that there is a place for using "SNAGS" in the pain free, seemingly mobile, direction. (When you manipulate a cervical spine it is usually done in the pain free direction). The procedure is exactly the same as for rotation to the restricted and painful side but you do not have the feedback from the patient which ensures you are on the correct segment.

(2). To increase side flexion and/or decrease the pain associated with this movement. (See figure 4)

The procedure is virtually the same as for rotation. The patient is seated. You stand behind the patient with your thumbs (as for rotation) over the spinous process of the vertebra above the suspected site. The patient slowly actively side flexes to the restricted and/or painful side and as the movement is felt to take place beneath the thumbs apply a sustained pressure up along the facet planes. It should not be painful. If it is you may not be on the correct level. With side flexion the vertebra tilts on the one beneath. You tilt your hands with it to ensure that as you push up, the upper facets move correctly.

Variations

As with rotation the technique can be applied unilaterally on an articular pillar. This is now what we usually do as the patients can effectively "SELF SNAG" over the spinous process for side flexion. (Described later). The other important feature is to have the patient apply side flexion overpressure with a hand pushing the head over. Remember to sustain this end range position for several seconds.

Figure 4

"SNAGS" for cervical side flexion. Patient can apply overpressure.

(3). To increase extension and /or decrease the pain associated with it. (See figure 5)

The procedure is almost identical to the two already described. The patient is seated and your thumbs are again used on the upper spinous process of the cervical segment involved. As the patient slowly extends his neck you push up along the facet treatment plane. Maintain this glide until the neck returns to the neutral position.

As will be repeated tediously over and over in this text no pain must be felt by the patient. If painful "SNAGS" would not be used. Remember to try more than one level if your first choice is painful. There is a tendency to locate on the spinous process below the appropriate one or rather this has often been so in my case. However a repositioning of my thumbs has brought those exclamations of agreeable surprise from the patient.

"SNAGS" for extension in the cervical spine will prove successful in more than 80% of patients. The technique is repeated several times and the movement reassessed. An important comment to make here is that when the neck moves into extension the facet joints now lie vertically. Allowances for this facet directional change must be made to ensure that you still glide up in the direction of the treatment plane.

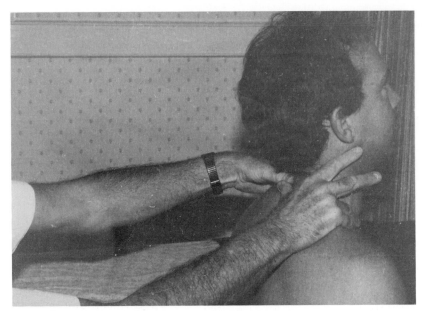

Figure 5

"SNAGS" for cervical extension

Variation

As the neck moves into extension the spinous processes approximate making it difficult to stay effectively on the chosen site. This is especially true if you have a small neck to work with and your thumbs are of a generous size. This is when "SELF SNAGS" are marvellous. They are so good in fact that in my practice nearly all patients with extension problems are immediately taught to "SELF SNAG". (Dealt with later).

(4). To increase flexion and/or decrease the pain associated with this movement.

There are two techniques that can dramatically improve a loss of flexion. The first to be briefly described is, as you would expect, "SNAGS" but the second is quite different and is called "FIST TRACTION".

"SNAGS" for flexion. (See figure 6)

You stand behind the seated patient and yes, one thumb reinforced by the other is placed over the superior spinous process of the spinal seg-

Figure 6

"SNAGS" for cervical flexion.

ment requiring therapy. As the patient flexes his neck slowly you push up along the treatment plane. In full flexion the treatment plane will be nearly horizontal and this directional change must be remembered or your mobilisation will be ineffective and probably painful. Several repetitions should bring results.

"FIST TRACTIONS" for flexion. (see figure 7)

These are ever so simple to do and in over 90% of patients who experience pain with neck flexion you will find them successful.

The patient is seated. Now place your clenched fist under his chin in the following manner. The point of the chin rests on the circular plateau formed by your curled index finger and thumb. Your curled little finger is placed on the upper edge of the sternum. The patient is asked to place one hand around the base of his occiput and pull the head forward and down. The chin cannot move due to the wedging effect of your fist which becomes a fulcrum for a skull rotation resulting in a distraction of the cervical spine. He would maintain this traction effect for ten seconds and repeat three times. It must not hurt. If it did you would try something else. Your fist must be large enough to limit any painful flexion from taking place. If a fist is small or the neck being treated large then pain will be felt before the chin meets the fist and thus the therapy will not work. A useful tip, in the case of a small hand, is to place the palm of the free hand on the patient's sternum under the little finger effectively providing a better fulcrum. Another alternative is to place a thick book under the chin as a wedge. Patient's should be taught and encouraged to apply self "FIST TRACTION" as a home program. They can use their own fist while pulling the head forward with their free hand or use a book as a wedge. With the latter they can then use both hands to apply the traction. They must always sustain the traction for at least ten seconds and repeat three times. "FIST TRACTIONS" are so good it is surprising that they were not thought of years ago.

If this technique does not work, and this is rare, the upper thoracic spine is probably where the problem lies. You would tend to suspect the upper thoracic spine if pain was only experienced with full neck flexion. A "SNAG" routine can be applied to this area. Stand behind the patient with your thumbs over the suspected thoracic vertebra's spinous process. As the patient flexes push up along the facet plane etc.

Figure 7
"FIST TRACTION" for a loss of flexion.

4. "SELF SNAGS"

Explanation

Manual therapy, be it manipulation or mobilisation, is normally undertaken to restore function and most therapists ask their patients to follow up the treatment with an exercise routine. In the case of the cervical spine we have found "SELF SNAGS" ever so useful as a home routine. In fact they can be so successful that it is often the only manual technique used when a patient presents for treatment. It is a revenue reducing technique as it tends to speed up a patient's recovery. Before showing the patient how to "SELF SNAG" I explain on an articulated spine what the procedure is all about. They can see for themselves the structures clearly and understand the purpose of the exercise.

Descriptions

(1). "SELF SNAGS" for cervical rotation. (See figure 8)

The only 'equipment' required is a small hand towel. The selvage on one side of the towel is hooked under the chosen spinous process. The ends of the towel on the same selvage side are firmly held by the patient with his forearms crossing. This would mean that one hand would lie above the other and the rule for the positioning is as follows. If the active movement required is right rotation then the right hand is on top holding the towel on the left side. The left hand (beneath) holds the towel on the right side. The left elbow is now hooked on the back of the chair to stabilise the arm and prevent thoracic rotation*. The right hand now pulls the towel up in the direction to the facet planes and then rotates the head to the right. When done properly the towel remains close to the side of the face. The upper right hand should position the towel so that it is close to the eye and keep it there as the movement takes place. As with "SNAGS" there must be no discomfort. If painful then try another level and check to ensure the direction of pull is accurate. As the arms are crossed the upper hand conveniently pulls the neck around. To enhance the therapy, rotation overpressure at end range can be applied by you the therapist or by someone in the patient's household. This assistance must not cause pain. After six to ten "SELF SNAGS" reassess and note the improvement. "SELF SNAGS" can be repeated two hourly initially if necessary. For left rotation the left hand would be on top to glide and guide the head around. We often get patients to "SELF SNAG" the incorrect level so that pain is felt with the movement. They then stop immediately and try other levels until they get it right.

Common mistakes that patients will make are . . .

(a) They forget to take their hands around with the head when turning. This will produce no relief from pain.

(b) They try to place a gathered towel under the spinous process instead of using the selvage. It is too bulky and not selective enough so that when they pull up, one facet does not specifically slide up on its inferior partner.

(c) Another error is to pull the towel forward and not up in the direction of the facet plane.

(d) Finally they forget to maintain the glide until the neck returns from its journey to the right or left. If the pressure is removed before the return to the midline a sharp pain can be felt. This is undesirable.

As with "SNAGS", there is a place for "SELF SNAGS" in the seemingly mobile pain free direction. However to be really useful overpressure at end range is essential. This means that assistance would be needed from a spouse or friend.

 * Hooking an elbow on the back of a chair was suggested by a New Zealand colleague (Zoe Clifford) and not mentioned in my earlier editions. There is no doubt that the by doing this the technique is much better and I now teach it this way on my courses.

(2). "SELF SNAGS" for side flexion or extension. (See figure 9)

As for rotation the patient is seated and a small towel is used. The selvage on one side is hooked under the spinous process of Cervical 5 if the offending segment is Cervical 5/6. The patient grips each end of the towel and pulls up along the treatment plane as he side flexes or extends his neck. When indicated the movement will increase and be pain free. It is repeated six to ten times and this routine could be undertaken every two hours or as you felt necessary. Pain and loss of extension is extremely common in patients presenting with cervical lesions. This "SELF SNAG" technique is so easy for the patient to do and so effective that in my practice it would be shown and used as a first step to improve extension instead of using "SNAGS". Remember to keep the towel in position as you extend to maintain the facet glide along the treatment plane.

Figure 8
"SELF SNAGS" for cervical rotation.

Figure 9

"SELF SNAGS" for cervical extension. The set up is exactly the same for side flexion.

5. SPINAL MOBILISATIONS WITH ARM MOVEMENT.
(SMWAMS)

Introduction

I guess this had to happen. Mobilisations with movement (MWMs) began in the spine when I developed "SNAGS" which of course are spinal mobilisations with spinal movements. From the spine I found they had an important role to play in the peripheral joints by combining extremity joint mobilisations with extremity joint movements. (you will read of these later in this book). What I have now found is that there is a place in manual therapy for combining a sustained spinal mobilisation with an extremity movement. In this section I will address their use in the upper extremity.

This new technique should be considered as a therapy when a patient presents with pain that is experienced with an upper extremity movement that could be of spinal origin.

Examples could be :

1. Pain radiating from the upper fibres of trapezius to the forearm when the arm is abducted above the horizontal.
2. Rhomboid pain felt by a patient when the arm is adducted across the body in the horizontal plane.
3. Pain radiating down to the hand with arm movements that involve the shoulder girdle.

This new mobilisation with movement developed because of the fact that when the shoulder girdle is moved, spinal movement also takes place because of the muscle attachments from the scapular to the cervical and upper thoracic vertebrae. You can prove this while reading. Place an index finger on say the spinous process of Cervical 7 and then move your free arm above the horizontal to involve the shoulder girdle. Agree?

This new technique is very simple to apply and should be used as part of your assessment as it has a diagnostic significance as well as being a therapy.

Description. (See figure 10)

To describe the basic technique let us assume your patient has pain radiating down to the flexor area of the left forearm when he horizontally adducts his shoulder.

You stand behind the seated patient. Because of the pain distribution, (Cervical 5) initially place your right thumb reinforced by the left over the left side of the patients 4th cervical vertebra. You now move the spinous process to the right and sustain this rotation as the patient horizontally adducts his left arm. If you are on the correct vertebra and the technique is appropriate the patient will feel no pain at all. After several repetitions the patient should then be able to move his arm in the offending direction without symptoms and without the accompanying sustained mobilisation . If this were not so then the treatment would be discarded. When successful two more sets of these pain free spinal mobilisations with arm movement (SMWAMS) would be undertaken.

Remember if there is any pain when the arm is moved do not proceed. Instead try the spinous process above or below your first choice in case you have chosen the incorrect level.

When the patient is moving his arm it is necessary that just enough momentum is used to ensure that a vertebral movement takes place at the segment you are trying to influence. Sensible patients can be taught to treat their own necks by placing a middle finger on the side of the vertebra and pulling it across as you did while they move the arm with the symptoms . The technique replicates what you did with them . They would

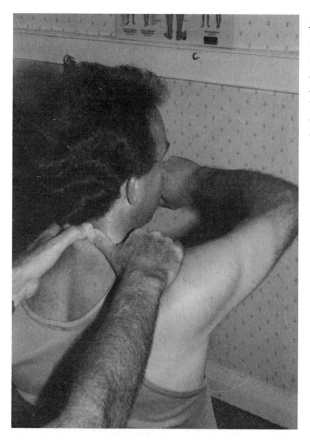

Figure 10

Spinal mobilisations with arm movement. In this case the spinous process of Cervical 4 is moved to the left with right horizontal adduction.

be instructed to repeat the therapy several times a day as you deem necessary. Another point to make is that the patient must hold his head in a good postural position while being treated. There is a tendency for the patient to flex his neck when your thumbs are positioned which tightens the posterior structures and makes your therapy ineffectual.

This technique can be used on the upper thoracic spine when the patient's upper thoracic pain is provoked with arm movement.

As with all MWMs it must be stressed that the glide in the chosen direction must not be released until the patient's arm returns to the starting position. This rule is very important.

Rationale

When you move, say the spinous process of Cervical 4 to the right, Cervical 4 rotates to the left on Cervical 5. This causes the facets of Cervical 4/5 on the left to separate and reposition. Now, when the left arm is raised above shoulder level, the muscle attachments from the scapular to the spine will make the Thoracic and Cervical vertebrae move, up to the level of the Cervical 4 vertebra which you have rotated to the left. At the level of Cervical 4/5 a mobilisation/ manipulation takes place that cannot be replicated by any other means. It causes a unique biomechanical effect which can prove extremely valuable therapeutically. Often an audible "click" can be heard similar to that which can be heard when you manipulate a facet joint.

Summary

These spinal mobilisations with arm movement are extremely effective when indicated, and thus really exciting and are completely safe if the basic rules are followed . These are:

1. When indicated no pain is experienced with the technique.

2. After six to ten repetitions of the arm movement with sustained spinal mobilisation the patient should notice a marked improvement in arm function. If not try another therapy.

3. Do not over treat. The quick change for the better in the status of the patient's symptoms may inspire the therapist to over treat. On day one if I have any concern about the patient I may only use one set of SMWAMS and review the patient a couple of days later.

4. As already stated do not release your mobilisation until the patient has returned to the starting position.

6. CERVICAL POSITIONAL SNAGS

Introduction

This I know is a most unusual heading but I cannot think of a better one and what I am about to describe must be included in this book . It is really a form of specific passive joint movement by you, the therapist, combined with an active movement and at this stage I am only using it for cervical rotation . The joints that really respond to it are at the Cervical 5/6 and 6/7 levels. I find the technique great for middle aged patients with some degenerative changes at these levels who present with a painful movement loss and where the pain they experience is not referred to the arm.

Figure 11

Cervical positional SNAGS. The patient pushes head further than the active range with a hand on the chin.

Description

We will assume that the patient has a painful loss of right rotation and his discomfort is felt in the adjacent muscles.

You stand behind the seated patient and place your right thumb to the right of the spinous process of Cervical 5 and your left thumb to the left of Cervical 6. (See figure 11). By moving your thumbs centrally you effect a rotation to the right of Cervical 5 on Cervical 6. Concurrently you ask the patient to actively rotate his head to the right. As with all "SNAGS" procedures the patient must experience no pain and to enhance the treatment have him push his head around further. (If there was pain with movement you may have chosen the wrong level). After six repetitions there should be improved function to the satisfaction of both you and the patient. If no change? Yes, you would try something else. Well done.

When the thumb pressure is uncomfortable push through some plastic foam .

B. THE UPPER CERVICAL SPINE - SPECIAL THERAPIES.

In this section I wish to deal with three specific conditions. They are "Acute Wry Neck, "Headaches" and "Vertigo".

1. THE ACUTE WRY NECK

In the May 1977 issue of the New Zealand Journal of Physiotherapy (3) I had an article published on this subject and since that time I have always used the method about to be described as it is always successful. We all know the condition is self limiting and will spontaneously recover in three or four days. The pain is unilateral, confined to the neck, is common in the young and is so distressing that patients usually seek medical attention. Because of the spasm encountered I consider manipulation unkind and unnecessary. The procedure I use is as follows.

The patient lies supine with his head on a pillow on which had been placed a hot pack or even a hot water bottle. He rests for a minute or two and then begins exercising his head in rotation to the painful restricted side. The range of movement is encouraged by small slow oscillations up to the pain block. It is a small teasing motion at the end of the range. Although discomfort is experienced it should never be so strong a movement as to be considered painful. Within five minutes of exercising the spasm slowly diminishes and the range of movement increases. In every case within twenty minutes (or less) a full range of movement will have returned. The patient will still experience pain with side flexion. On standing the neck will still be painful but much better. He should rest that day and not return to work or school. We tell them when they get home to put on a folded pillowcase collar. Before going off to sleep that night I suggest they remove the collar, lie with the head on a pillow and repeat the exercise routine that they undertook in my clinic. The collar is then replaced for the night. The next morning they can expect to be 90% better. Rarely do we have to see them twice. If this form of therapy did not work I would respectfully suggest that the patient does not have an Acute Wry Neck. Remember that a wry neck does not produce a headache, there are no radicular signs and the pain is unilateral.

2. HEADACHES

Explanation

The treatments for patients plagued by headaches has been of special interest to me for over two decades. However I will confine comments on this subject to my special tests and treatments for this condition and a "SNAGS" technique that we find useful in restoring a loss of Cervical 1/2 (atlas/axis) rotation which is often associated with a headache.

If a patient is suffering from a headache of upper cervical origin then one of the mobilisations or the traction to be described should, as it is being applied, stop the pain. They are sustained techniques. I assume that if a headache stops with a technique involving the upper cervical spine then this must be diagnostically significant as to the site of the lesion causing the problem.

The first technique is like the "NAGS" mobilisations already covered but differs in that the top two vertebrae are moved ventrally on the base of the stationary occiput above.

The second is where the occiput is drawn forward on the upper cervical spine.

The third is a form of manual traction which distracts the upper cervical facets at right angles to their treatment planes.

The fourth as already mentioned is a mobilisation with movement that can restore a loss of Cervical 1/2 rotation.

Descriptions

(1). "HEADACHE SNAGS". (See figures 12a and b)

You stand beside the seated patient. His head is cradled between your body and the right forearm if you stand on his right side. (See earlier description of head position for "NAGS"). The right index and middle finger wrap around the base of the occiput and the middle phalanx of the little finger lies over the spinous process of Cervical 2. (It is prominent and is the first process palpable about 2.5cms below the occiput). The left thenar eminence lies over the right little finger. Pressure is now applied in a ventral direction on the spinous process of Cervical 2 while the skull remains still due to the control of your right forearm. The gentle moving force to do this comes from your left arm via the thenar eminence over the little finger on the spine of Cervical 2. The first thing that happens is that the second vertebra moves forward on the first until the slack is taken up then the first vertebra moves forward on the base of the skull. This is quietly taken forward until end range is felt and this position

Figure 12a
"HEADACHE SNAGS"

        Figure 12b
        "SELF HEADACHE SNAGS"

is maintained for at least ten seconds. If indicated the headache will lift and you have two ways now to deal with it. The first is for you to manually repeat the "HEADACHE SNAGS" six to ten times. The second is to have the patient "SELF HEADACHE SNAG" . This is achieved by placing the now familiar hand towel around the spinous process of Cervical 2 and securing it with the hands. The patient now glides his head back without tilting it which will replicate what you the therapist did with the "HEADACHE SNAG". This is not a strong procedure as excessive muscle activity between the occiput and the spine would be counterproductive. The patient sustains the posterior glide for at least ten seconds and repeats the process six to ten times. They should now feel much better. The technique can be repeated as often as you feel necessary during the day. Remember that the facet planes we are dealing with here lie in an antero-posterior direction and do not slope upwards like their lower relations.

"Woolly head" sensation. If patients experience what they describe as a woolly sensation in the head after an upper cervical manipulation "HEADACHE SNAGS" should be used. These will often, after a few repetitions, rid the patients of their distress.

(2). "REVERSE HEADACHE SNAGS" . (See figure 13)

The patient is seated with the head held in the manner described previously except that the right little finger is wrapped around the base of the occiput and makes no contact with the cervical spine. The thumb and index finger of the left hand wrap around Cervical 2 so that the web between them is in contact with the posterior part of the neck. The spine is thus held securely but the grip should be comfortable and care taken not to "throttle" the patient. While the upper cervical spine is stabilised in this manner, the head is taken forward on the column to end range and held there for at least ten seconds. In moving the skull you must not tilt it to ensure that the facet planes remain parallel. If this technique is indicated the headache will go and several repeat mobilisations should be undertaken. As you will have noted this technique is the reverse of the previous one. A Sydney colleague suggested when I was teaching recently that the same effect could perhaps be achieved by the patient, if he were to wrap a towel around his occiput to stabilise it, and then glide his neck posteriorly. I would agree. Self "FIST TRACTION" are often useful when patients respond to "REVERSE HEADACHE SNAGS".

(3). UPPER CERVICAL TRACTION (See figures 14a and b)

For many headaches, that are the result of a biomechanical problem in the upper cervical spine, traction in slight extension is the treatment of choice. Remember when dealing with facet joints any traction being ap-

Figure 13

"REVERSE HEADACHE SNAGS"

plied must take place at right angles to the treatment plane. The testing technique to be described complies with this rule when applying a distraction to the atlanto-occipital and atlas-axis joints.

The patient lies supine and you place the lower section of your right (or left) forearm under his cervical spine so that the ventral border of your radius is tucked under the base of his occiput. If you have a small forearm, or perhaps the patient is large, you can place a narrowly folded towel under your arm to raise it a little. Now place two fingers of your other hand under his chin. To apply traction pronate the forearm tucked under the occiput while delivering an equal pressure under the chin with your fingers. The effect will be a distraction of the upper cervical joints while the natural lordosis is maintained due to the positioning of the forearm. Hold the traction for at least ten seconds and see if the headache goes. Very little distraction is needed and care must be taken to ensure that the occipital and chin forces equate or the head will tilt and the desired effect will be lost. Experience has shown me that over 90% of headaches of upper cervical origin that I see cease while this type of traction is being applied. On this basis alone it is worth trying. When effective it is easy to set up a sustained traction treatment using a cervical harness, a small weight and supporting the lordosis with a rolled up towel.

Figure 14a
Upper cervical traction. Test and treatment.

Figure 14b
Upper cervical traction in extension with harness. Note rolled towel.

(4). "SNAGS" for restricted Cervical 1/2 rotation. (See figure 15a)

This technique can be extremely useful in restoring upper cervical rotation and especially when manipulation is contraindicated or the therapist does not have manipulative skills. Most patients can be taught to "SELF SNAG" which is a bonus.

The patient is seated and you stand behind him. Let us assume he has lost right Cervical 1/2 rotation. You place the pad of the terminal phalanx of your left thumb as far laterally as you can on the transverse process of Cervical 1 on the left. This is large and readily palpated just below the occiput. Your right thumb is now placed over its partner. The patient is asked to slowly rotate his head to the right while you provide a gliding force ventrally on Cervical 1 with your thumbs to assist the movement. As the head rotates your thumbs must move around with it to remain on "target". There must be no pain as is the rule for all "SNAG" techniques. Remember that the treatment plane at this level is almost horizontal when the patient is seated. Thumb pressure is not released until the neck returns to the mid line. If this did not work then you would "SNAG" on the other side with rotation to the right.

"SELF SNAGS". For these a small towel is required, as was the case with the other cervical joints already dealt with. The selvage on one side is placed around the back of the neck immediately below the occiput so that it lies over Cervical 1. For left rotation the patient holds the towel on the right with his left hand and the end of the towel on the left with his right hand. The left hand should lie above the right. The right elbow would be hooked on the back of the chair. As the patient turns his head around to the left his left hand assists Cervical 1 to rotate by pulling it round. (See figure 15b). It must not hurt. If it proves successful the patient can be instructed to repeat sets of six frequently during the day or as you think fit.

This "SELF SNAG" becomes even more effective if the patient gets his partner to apply overpressure to the movement. The overpressure should produce no discomfort.

Figure 15a

"SNAGS" for restricted rotation at Cervical 1/2.

Figure 15b

"SELF SNAGS" for restricted rotation at Cervical 1/2.

(3). VERTIGO AND OTHER VERTEBRAL ARTERY SIGNS

Explanation

Vertebral artery signs are a contraindication to manipulation and all manual therapists are aware of the protocols that exist to test for these signs. However there are simple mobilisations with movement that you can do which will often bring about a safe resolution to the patient's problem. This treatment is only applied for the vertigo or other signs that are produced with neck movement and it is usually neck extension that most commonly causes giddiness. However rotation can also be a problem as can flexion. I have yet to see a patient that experiences vertigo etc. with both left and right rotation even though they may have symptoms with both flexion and extension movements.

Description

Before the treatment is tried you must ensure that you have the full co-operation of the patient. He will be asked to move his head in the direction that produces his symptoms, provided that with mobilisation this movement is symptom free. He STOPS if it produces giddiness or other vertebral artery signs. As with all "SNAGS" techniques they are only used if they are symptom free. If you follow this rule you will never exacerbate a patient's condition.

If extension causes the problem you stand behind the seated patient. Place the palmar aspect of the first phalanx of one thumb reinforced by the other over the spinous process of Cervical 2. You now push ventrally as the patient slowly extends his neck. When indicated the patient will be able to extend his neck symptom free. The forward thumb pressure is sustained until the neck returns to the starting position. Repeat the mobilisation with movement six times. The patient should now be able to extend his neck without experiencing vertigo or nausea. That would be all you would do by way of manual therapy on day one.

(Perhaps in this text it should be mentioned that patients who have problems with their necks in bed should be supplied with a soft collar to sleep in. In my practice we advise patients to fold an empty pillow case in half longways and then into three and wrap it around the neck securing it with a safety pin. It is amazing how effective the pillow case is.)

If the patient is reasonably intelligent you would show him how to "SELF SNAG" his neck so that the treatment can be repeated several times a day should this be necessary. The procedure with the small towel is the same as for a loss of neck extension. However you keep the towel parallel with the upper jaw as you move into extension because of the treatment plane. Some patients only require one treatment, others may require three or four but when this technique is indicated and used the patient always makes a rapid recovery.

If right rotation is the offending movement you have three thumb positional choices.

(1). Start over the spinous process of Cervical 2 as you did for extension. As the patient rotates to the side that produces his symptoms you again push ventrally remembering to follow the process as it moves away from the mid line. If indicated and done correctly the vertigo will not appear. If it does, do not proceed. Instead try your second choice.

(2). On this occasion place your thumb reinforced by the other on the end of the transverse process of Cervical 1 on the left side. It is easy to palpate just below the occiput. As the patient rotates in the offending direction you push the articular pillar forward with your thumbs, being mindful of the treatment plane. If symptoms appear STOP.

(3). Repeat the rotation with your thumbs on the right side. I have found that when the patient has "vertebral artery" signs with rotation, movement with mobilisation on the contralateral side has been the most successful.

The reader will note that we used these techniques to restore Cervical 1/2 rotation.

When one of the above proves to be successful repeat the manoeuvre six times. The patient should now experience a marked improvement when he rotates his head. Remember that visual disturbances associated with neck movement can also respond to these techniques.

Since using these mobilisations with movements we have only had one patient who has not responded to them in the last three years.

We even succeeded in stopping one patient from refluxing every time he rotated his head to the right. (Socially embarrassing?) The symptoms had been with him for over nine months and only three treatments were necessary. One year later he was still symptom free. Physiotherapy really does get more satisfying as the years pass.

Why do these techniques work? The explanation that I give to my patients is that their vertigo is due to a gliding malfunction in one or more of the joints in the upper cervical spine. The easiest way to show this to them is to use an articulated spine.

C. THE LUMBAR SPINE

1. "SNAGS"

Introduction

"SNAGS" in the treatment of the lumbar spine added a new dimension to my therapies for this area. They have proved so exciting to use when indicated and because of this some theorising became inevitable when wondering how a procedure can be so useful. However we all know that it is unwise to print one's theories because if they can be faulted the author's credibility is questioned and any valid treatment claims made could be cast aside. Anyway the reader may find my following comments of interest.

Different manual therapy schools of thought have thrived through the decades with their respective followers and this has bothered those of us with orthodox minds. We read of facet theories, disc theories, muscle theories and so on. Today gaining scientific acceptance is the McKenzie (2) treatment approach which fits in so neatly with the disc theory. Up until now one thing has always puzzled me about the disc theory. This has been the fact that a simple facet manipulation can sometimes bring great relief to a patient that we "know" has a disc lesion. I will now offer one hypothesis which I feel ties in facet hypomobility with disc involvement. It explains why "SNAGS", which I believe work directly on facet joints, can help a disc lesion and certainly assist with the response to a McKenzie (2) or other routine. These remarks definitely pertain to the lumbar spine.

During normal flexion of the spine the disc distorts and becomes wedge shaped. The vertebral bodies proximate ventrally and separate dorsally. The nucleus (or whatever) moves posteriorly, but the disc whose volume is unalterable, remains under the umbrella of the vertebra above. (See figure 16). For this to occur the facets joints must be mobile. If the facet joints are hypomobile, when flexion takes place, the vertebral bodies will be able to proximate anteriorly but unable to separate dorsally. The disc may no longer remain under the umbrella of the vertebra above and instead bulge posteriorly causing symptoms. These symptoms would all be a matter of degree. If there was a weakness in the posterior wall of the disc then even greater problems would arise from facet hypomobility. What I am implying is that most back pain comes from the disc which is producing symptoms due in no small measure to the facets. When you have a patient, who has pain to the lateral lower leg with spinal flexion standing, and you "SNAG" him, and while doing so his leg pain disappears, you will probably support my hypothesis.

As with all techniques an explanation must be given to the patients. This is really important in the lumbar spine as a lack of understanding could lead to an exacerbation of their pain and without their co-operation the procedures will not work. You tell patients that you are going to move a vertebra with your hand in such a way that the pain they feel with a particular movement will disappear. If they feel any pain they must tell you so that you can check your technique or try another level. Without their help "SNAGS" are valueless. I must say at this point, do not overdo the "SNAGS". As soon as an improvement is brought about on day one stop and see them two days later. As a matter of fact we now teach " the rule of three". On day one when treating a patient with marked pain and thus distress we only use our pain free techniques three times as a precaution. This way you cannot exacerbate a patient. Too much enthusiasm can leave them sore the next day. We are all aware of the latent effects that any manual therapy can have.

If no change is elicited then "SNAGS" are inappropriate. You expect an immediate improvement. Remember that other physiotherapy should also be given and as I stated in the introduction to Part One you should use the McKenzie approach when a patient has a Lumbar 4/5 lesion with a lateral shift.

In treating the cervical and upper thoracic spines with "SNAGS" the patient is seated on a chair. For the lumbar, middle and lower thoracic spines we require a plinth and a belt that can be adjusted in length. The belt needs to be 2.6 metres (8 feet) in length and made from car seatbelt material with a suitable easy to release clasp. As will become apparent it makes the patient stable while mobilisations with movement are carried out.

The techniques will now be described as they would be applied for movements in the lumbar spine that are painful and/or restricted. When assessing your patients' active movements for restrictions and/or pain you should do this in both sitting and standing. If their movement problems are only present when standing then "SNAGS" are only done in standing. If they have movement problems when sitting as well then your initial therapy would be in sitting and would progress to standing.

As with the cervical spine many patients, when taught, can apply "SELF SNAGS" and this will be covered at the end of this section.

Figure 16

Anterior

Posterior

DISC

VERT 1

VERT 2

*With normal flexion discal
content is displaced from the
anterior of the disc (=a) and
is accommodated posteriorly
disc (=b)*

Normal
Flexion

Posterior

Anterior

VERT 1

VERT 2

b *a*

Anterior

Abnormal flexion

Posterior

VERT 1

?b *a*

VERT 2

*If facets are locked or
hypomobile the vetebral
bodies can proximate
anteriorly but posteriorly are
unable to separate. There is
an abnormal discal bulge (?b)
or unacceptable pain
producing pressure on the
posterior disc wall.*

Descriptions

(1). To increase flexion and/or decrease the pain associated with this movement.

a. In sitting.

The patient sits over the edge of a plinth. You stand behind and place a belt around him and yourself as shown in Figure 17a. In placing the belt around the patient's lower abdomen keep it below the anterior superior iliac spines for comfort. The belt should be at the level of your sacrum or lower. The ulnar border of your right hand is now placed under the spinous process of the vertebra above at the suspected spinal segment. The patient flexes forward until the pain is felt. He now backs off a little from this position. You now apply a gliding force up along the treatment plane as he again flexes. If the treatment is indicated, you are on the right segment and the direction of force is correct, he will painlessly flex to almost full range. If there is pain try another level. Sustain this flexed position for a few seconds and maintain your facet pressure until the patient is again erect. Failure to maintain the glide could lead to a sharp and unnecessary pain. When there is no pain, repeat just three times and that would be all that you would do on the patient's first visit. If this central "SNAG" is not helpful a unilateral glide should be tried. Let us assume your patient has a Lumbar 4/5 segmental lesion. To do this place the ulnar border of your right hand (just distal to the pisaform) over the articular pillar of Lumbar 4 on the right. As the patient flexes push up along the facet plane. If unsuccessful try a unilateral "SNAG" on the opposite side. With the passage of time I tend to use the unilateral "SNAG" rather than the central.

Instead of the ulnar border of the hand the thumbs can be used when dealing with Lumbar 4/5 and lumbosacral levels. As with the cervical spine one thumb reinforces the other which is placed over the chosen superior facet. (See figure 17b). They glide the superior facet up as flexion takes place. N.B. It is impossible to use your thumbs above Lumbar 4/5 as the inferior facet projects posteriorly further than its partner making correct thumb contact impossible.

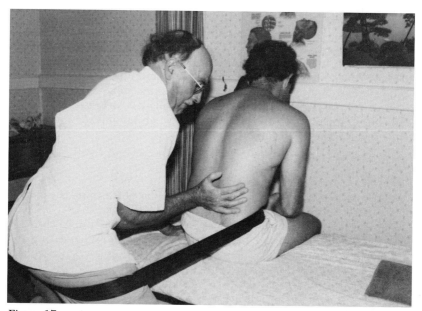

Figure 17a

"SNAGS" for lumbar flexion in sitting.

Figure 17b

"SNAGS" for lumbar flexion using thumbs over left lumbar 5 facet.

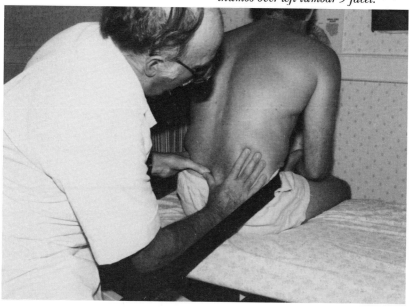

Important

When treating a patient who presents with an acute lumbar lesion and responds immediately to flexion "SNAGS", stop after three repetitions and tape the spine in hyperextension to prevent further aggravation. Two strips of 2.5 centimetre adhesive tape used diagonally across the lumbar spine are extremely effective. We would of course encourage extensions as they would be taught by physiotherapists using R A McKenzie's protocols (3). At this juncture I would add one proviso and that is we would avoid extension if it were painful.

b. In standing.

With the patient standing, place the now familiar belt around the patient and yourself as it was when the patient was seated. (See figure 18). "SNAGS" are now undertaken in the same way as they were in sitting. However have the patient slightly flex his knees as this will remove hamstring and sciatic nerve tension facilitating a better response. Remember as with all "SNAGS" techniques maintain your pressure until the patient is erect again. It may be necessary to "SNAG" unilaterally as suggested when the patient is sitting and this is done in exactly the same way. The patients' response is often improved if they are close to a table or bed on which they can place a hand for stability.

Figure 18

"SNAGS" for lumbar flexion in standing.

(2). To increase extension and/or decrease the pain associated with this movement.

If extension is painful and limited in sitting then you would start with the patient sitting on the plinth with his legs over the side. You stand behind the patient with the belt around you both. I find it easier to have it lower on me as you will see in Figure 19. The ulnar border of your right (or left) hand is placed under the superior spinous process of the vertebral segment involved. Providing he feels no pain the patient extends his lumbar spine while you push up along the treatment plane. If you study the photograph of this technique you will note that I am standing slightly to one side to ensure I am not in the patient's way as he extends. His co-operation is essential. If painful he must stop and you would try another level. If still painful try "SNAGGING" over the articular pillar on the right or perhaps the left.

N.B. A problem encountered with some patients is that they lean back against your hand instead of extending their lumbar spines. This is terrible as you take all the upper body weight and feel that your wrist may brake. See that they get it right!

We all see many patients with chronic low back pain who on examination have painful limited extension and apparent normal pain free flexion. What is often necessary with these sufferers if "SNAGS" for extension is unsuccessful, is to "SNAG" them in flexion first. This would appear to release the facet(s) at the offending level and make a spectacular difference when "SNAGS" are again repeated for extension.

As with the "SNAGS" technique for flexion you would progress to the standing position. Standing would of course be the starting position if extension in sitting was symptomless in the first place. (See figure 20)

When "SNAGS" for extension are indicated repeat the mobilisation with movement only three or four times on day one. The patient should now be able to extend unassisted and without pain. More "SNAGS" may be required but do not over treat. Some patients feel some discomfort the next day but if the rules with regard to pain are followed no problems will be encountered. If the articular pillar on one side is being chosen for extension select the side of pain first. This technique can be a strain on the therapist. To minimize this, tuck the elbow of the mobilising arm into the waist and keep the leg on this side well behind you for stability.

QUESTION?

When teaching "SNAGS" for extension, physiotherapists often ask for an explanation as to why I glide the superior facet up for extension when it allegedly is supposed to slide down. I have two theories to offer. The first is that the superior facet is "jammed" down on its partner and extension

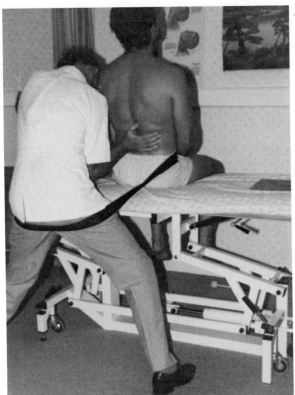

Figure 19
"SNAGS" for lumbar extension in sitting.

Figure 20
"SNAGS" for lumbar extension in standing.

Manual Therapy

"jams" it further. Pushing it up before extension takes place re- positions it to enable it to now behave biomechanically as it was designed to. The second is that with extension the top vertebra rotates slightly in the sagittal plane. Pushing up through the spinous process assists this rotation. I guess the point is they work when indicated and that is all that matters.

(3). To increase rotation and/or decrease the pain associated with this movement.

The patient sits astride one end of the plinth facing the other end. This stabilises the pelvis which is important. He places his hands behind his neck. Let us assume the patient has a painful loss of right rotation resulting from a lesion at the Lumbar 2/3 level. You stand behind the patient and wrap your right arm around him clasping the side just above the suspected level of the lesion. (See figure 21). The ulnar border of your left hand is placed under the spinous process of Lumbar 2. The patient

Figure 21
"SNAGS" for lumbar or thoracic rotation.

now rotates to the right as your left hand "SNAGS" the segment. There must be no pain. Your right hand around the waist encourages the movement and can apply overpressure when indicated. To this end your hand around the waist must be above the level of the segment being treated or it will be unable to apply overpressure. If this procedure is ineffective you can next try "SNAGS" over the articular pillar on the right or left. To do this use the pisaform area of the hand to effect the glide. If the elbow of the mobilising arm rests in the ventral fold of your hip joint then an upward glide of your pelvis will assist with the facet glide. It is similar to a "bedroom" manoeuvre that would be familiar to a few readers. It is not however reproductive - it should produce no pain.

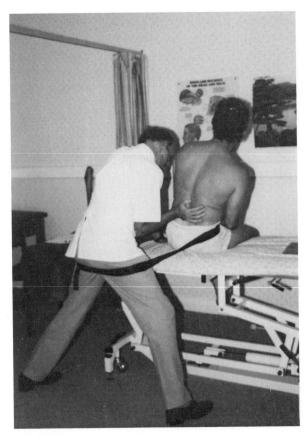

Figure 22

"SNAGS" for lumbar side flexion in sitting.

(4). To increase side flexion and/or decrease the pain associated with this movement.

"SNAGS" are really useful for a side flexion loss. Even if you have a patient with a lateral shift that is proving recalcitrant try restoring side flexion in the manner to be described. The patient sits on the side of the bed with his back to you. A belt is around you both as demonstrated in Figure 22. For a loss of right side flexion place the ulnar border of your right hand over the appropriate spinous process as has now been described many times. You would stand slightly to the left of the patient. The belt would then serve to stabilise the patient as he side flexes while you are gliding the superior facet up. Active pain free movement can be expected if the technique is correct and you have chosen the correct level. You could repeat this mobilisation with movement six times and that would be sufficient on the first visit.

This technique can be applied in standing if thought necessary though it is more difficult on the operator.

As with all the previous treatments that have been covered you may have to "SNAG" over an articular pillar.

2. "SELF SNAGS"

Explanation and Description

As with the cervical spine it is possible for many patients to "SELF SNAG" their lumbar spines particularly for flexion and extension and sometimes for side flexion. I would like here to refer to the repeated extensions in standing recommended by McKenzie (2). These are encouraged for instance if they centralise a pain that is experienced in the posterior thigh. When a belt is used successfully by the patient to "SELF SNAG" they can do repeated extensions in standing painlessly and after several repetitions actively extend without the belt painlessly. The purpose of "SNAGS" is to bring about an immediate improvement in the patient's movement after they have been completed. To successfully "SNAG" a joint several times and find that there is no change following their application would also suggest that the treatment is inappropriate.

The patient requires a belt, (ideally of car seat belt material or soft leather), that is long enough to pass around his back and still be held at short arm's length away from his body on each side. (See figure 23a).

If the segmental lesion is at Lumbar 3/4 then the belt is hooked under the spinous process of Lumbar 3.

Extension is the most commonly used "SELF SNAG". As the patient moves into spinal extension he pulls up on the belt in the direction of his chin and if no pain is experienced this is repeated say six times and then two hourly or as you think necessary. Another method is to have the patient clench a fist and place the shaft of the first phalanx of his index finger under the spinous process. With the assistance of his other hand he pushes up along the treatment plane as he extends. For unilateral "SELF SNAGS" again a fist is used. This time the flexed metacarpo-phalangeal joint of the index finger is placed over the articular pillar on one side. (See figure 23b). As said before an articulated spine is a wonderful asset to use when trying to explain to a patient where to push and of course to explain what the technique is all about.

It helps if the patient is intelligent and has reasonably strong arms.

"SELF SNAGS" for flexion are accomplished in the same way as for extension. However as with "SNAGS" have the patient slightly flex his knees to ease the tension on the hamstrings and sciatic nerve.

Warning. If flexion is limited and the patient is in a great deal of pain, "SELF SNAGS" for flexion would be inadvisable until with your management they feel more comfortable.

The common fault that we encounter with "SELF SNAGS" is where the patient does not pull up along the treatment plane as the movement takes place. He starts off correctly but forgets to raise his arms as he goes back. Another problem is that he releases the pull up before he returns to the upright position. "SELF SNAGS" with a belt for the lumbo-sacral joint will not work if the patient's posterior iliac borders protrude further posteriorly than Lumbar 5's spinous process. The edge of the belt cannot physically make contact with it.

Figure 23a

"SELF SNAGS" for lumbar extension with a belt.

Figure 23b

"SELF SNAGS" for lumbar extension using hands.

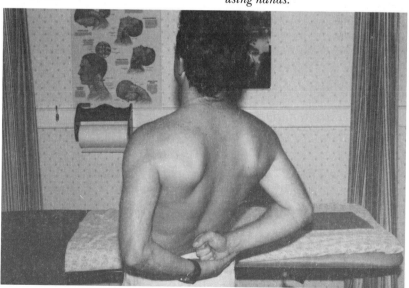

D. THE THORACIC SPINE

"SNAGS"

Explanation and Descriptions.

As the reader would expect the techniques for the thoracic spine are really the same as those for the lumbar spine. In practice the most useful "SNAG" is the one for rotation as this is the movement most commonly requiring attention in patients with thoracic lesions.

(1). To restore rotation and/or decrease the pain associated with this movement.

The patient positioning and technique is the same as that for lumbar rotation. The difficulty is with large patients particularly women. The problem, if you have short arms, comes when you try to wrap your arm around the patient to clasp the side just above the suspected level. (Refer figure 21).

Experience will show you that unilateral positioning is required more frequently than centrally over the spinous process. Do not over "SNAG". As soon as a marked improvement is obtained stop. Quite often with thoracic lesions you need to deal with both right and left rotation and you would do this on day one if both were involved. After restoring pain free rotation I always then support the thoracic spine for 48 hours with two short pieces of 5 centimetre wide zinc oxide tape placed diagonally across the site of the lesion.

(2). To restore flexion and/or decrease the pain associated with this movement.

The patient sits astride the plinth as for rotation. If you are standing behind and to his right, place your right arm around his trunk at the level of the lesion. This is used as a fulcrum for bending. Your left hand's ulnar border is placed over the selected spinous process or articular pillar and supplies the gliding force along the facet plane as the patient flexes. (See figure 24)

Figure 24

"SNAGS" for thoracic flexion in sitting.

(3). To restore extension and/or decrease the pain associated with it.

In the lower thoracic spine the "SNAGS" procedure is the same as that used for the lumbar spine. (Using belt).

For the mid thoracic spine the patient sits astride the plinth with you at his side. As you will see from Figure 25, one hand is applying the "SNAGS" while the free arm is wrapped around the patient guiding the movement. Some strength is required to support the patient during extension as well as providing the facet glide. It is easier to have the flexed elbow of the arm responsible for the "SNAGS" tucked into your side. This would be the most physically demanding of all the "SNAGS" techniques. Thank goodness that this technique is rarely required. As already stated rotation techniques are generally used in the thoracic spine.

Figure 25
"SNAGS" for thoracic
extension in stride sit-
ting.

E. CONCLUSION

All the "NAGS" and "SNAGS" techniques described in this section on the spine are basic ones. Once they are mastered therapists adapt them to their own requirements. This may be necessary because of different body types. I use many starting variations but the principles are not altered. Some patients present with more than one level of involvement and this requires some imagination to deal with. I have even combined them with a slump stretch and when next you get a patient with a limited straight leg raise, and apparent normal spinal movement, "SNAG" for flexion over Lumbar 5 or perhaps Lumbar 4 and see what happens when you retest. When next you have a patient with a persistent hamstring lesion try a lumbo-sacral "SNAGS" and see if this "fixes" the problem.

One difficulty encountered but easily solved is due to perspiration particularly in hot climates. If either the patient's or your skin is moist then slipping will occur particularly with "SNAGS". This can be overcome by the judicious use of a paper tissue. (eg Kleenex or Snowtex)

If you abide by the rules no complications will arise and remember, do not do too much on the patient's first visit.

2. OTHER SPINAL THERAPIES

A. Manipulation

I would support those that claim that manipulations are much more useful in the treatment programs for the cervical and upper thoracic spines than in the management of lumbar and lower thoracic lesions. This is because the facet joints are probably more directly responsible for pain emanating from the cervical spine. Physiotherapists should read "Where Is The Pain Coming From" by V. Mooney published in "Spine" in 1987.(4)

In my preamble on "SNAGS" at the beginning of the section on the lumbar spine I wrote of the need to have mobile facets for normal discal distortions to take place with spinal movement. What happens when we manipulate a lumbar spinal joint? We hear and feel a click. Most practitioners agree that this is usually a facet sound. Some patients feel instantly better but others say it has made no difference even though you are sure the correct segment has been dealt with. I would say with the former the manipulation has enabled the facet joints to glide normally removing the abnormal strain on the disc. With the latter the joints, though manipulatively gapped, are still unable to perform normally. To use "SNAGS" makes sense but there are patients who fail to respond to these but will do so after a preceding manipulation. The danger from manipulation as I see it is from manipulating with the "wrong side up". Strict guidelines cannot be given. If the incorrect side is chosen too much unnatural torsional strain can be placed on a weakened disc. It is not until after your manipulation that you find you have worsened the disc pathology. Dangers are minimised by skilled manipulators who, because of their technical ability, use minimal force when thrusting. However "SNAGS" are much safer.

B. Belt traction techniques

The belt I use for "SNAGS" to the lumbar spine and adequately described in earlier text can be used to apply traction to many segments of the spine. I had an article published on this subject in Gregory Grieve's magnificent tome "Modern Manual Therapy of the Vertebral column".(5)

In the preface I mentioned how techniques change for the better as time passes. This is certainly true of a technique described in my paper in Greg Grieve's book. It relates to the application of traction to the middle and lower thoracic and lumbar spines. Although as explained it achieves a successful distraction the strain on the therapist is considerable. I have thus modified the procedure to avoid this and enable those of smaller stature to cope. The belt tractions for the cervical spine I have not had to alter.

For the mid-thoracic to the low lumbar spine have the patient lying supine on a plinth covered with non slip material. The plinth should be on carpeted floor to prevent it from moving when the patient is tractioned and be adjustable in height for convenience.

The belt is positioned under the spinous process of the vertebra above the offending segment and its loop encircles your shoulders. (See figure 26). The patient needs to place his hands around your waist when dealing with the mid thoracic spine to move the scapulae laterally on the chest wall. A pillow may be placed under the head. The reader will see from Figure 26 that the therapist's hips are slightly flexed so that his trunk hovers over the patient's body. You place your hands on the plinth with bent arms. The hands will become a fulcrum for a movement about to take place. You now extend your arms to secure the belt at the chosen level and by leaning backwards and pivoting on the fully extended arms you will traction the spine distal to the belt. Making use of the arms in this way ensures that no stress is placed on your spine and this is important. I have seen small therapists apply extremely effective traction on large patients without effort in this way. The use of belts to apply traction to the vertebral column has introduced a hitherto unobtainable degree of specificity and make manual traction so easy.

Traction applied in this manner would be sustained for more than ten seconds and can be repeated and repeated over many minutes. If it produced any pain you would not use it. If a patient was experiencing thoracic pain with breathing it should not be present when the distraction is taking place and after several repetitions should have disappeared altogether. Patients with anterior thigh pain radiating from lumbar 2/3 should experience relief when traction is applied with the belt hooked on lumbar 2. Thoracic manipulations are much easier to do after traction has been locally applied. A good follow up home traction will be described next.

C. Self tractions for the mid and lower thoracic and lumbar spines

This technique is invaluable for acute pain of spinal origin especially from the thoracic spine. With those patients who experience chest pain with breathing, relief is nearly always obtained. The procedure is simple and it is the time factor that makes it work.

The patient stands beside a table of suitable height or the back of a chair or whatever. He places his hands on the table so that the distance between them is greater than the width of the hips. Keeping his elbows locked in extension he bends his knees and allows the body to sink. In this position the shoulders would be elevated, the flexed toes only would be on the floor and the front of the body would be against the table. Seen from the side, the head, shoulders and hips would be in a vertical line

Figure 26

Belt traction for the mid thoracic to lower lumbar spine.

with the knees slightly forward of this. (See figure 27). If the knees are placed behind the trunk, traction would not take place. Instead a form of extension would result and this would be useless.

Patients must maintain this position for at least 20 seconds. By this time any thoracic pain being experienced would have stopped. If not, check the position to ensure it is correct. With the patients I spoke of with pain on inspiration, you should find that it has disappeared by the 20 seconds. If the correct technique does not relieve the pain then forget it. Try something else. In my practice I tell young patients that they are expected to self traction for 30 seconds three times and repeat this routine every two hours. Older patients are asked to self traction for 20 seconds three times and repeat this routine every two hours if they can manage it.

This form of self traction is a useful "first aid" measure for patients smitten with sudden back pain.

Note! When standing up after self traction patients must take care not to flex the spine as this could spoil the therapy. To avoid this after the sustained traction they bring one foot forward so that it lies beneath them. They use this leg to stand straight up.

Another very good way of doing this is between the backs of two chairs. (See figure 28) The hands clasp the adjacent chair backs and with the elbows straight bend you knees as above. It is hard on the palms of some patients and to get chair backs of suitable height is the other problem.

Important! The next four techniques to be described are extremely important and are used daily in my practice, when Straight Leg Raising is involved, to see if one of them has a role to play as a treatment. In fact one of them is usually proved effective. The first two have the added advantage of being useful as a home treatment by the patient. The second two are invaluable but not as a self treatment and thus not revenue reducing. After these I will discuss sitting and a simple new chair design which modesty prevents me from saying is very very good.

Figure 27

Self traction for the thoracic and lumbar spines.

Figure 28
Self traction for the thoracic spine between two chairs.

D. The bent leg raise technique

This is a painless technique, when indicated, and can be tried on any patient with low back pain who has limited and/or painful straight leg raising (SLR). It can be tried even if they have leg pain and can be extremely useful when you are confronted with one of those patients who has a gross bilateral limitation of straight leg raising. You will never make them worse if the absence of pain when applying your technique is your guide. If the bent leg raise (BLR) cannot be executed without pain then it is not to be used. The same rule as for "SNAGS". As with the techniques already covered in this book you do not over treat on the patient's first visit and we now teach the "rule of three" which means on day one the technique would only be used three times as a precaution against any latent exacerbation. We would try this technique on nearly every patient we see and it proves of great value with more than half of them. Remember it must not hurt.

You stand at the limited SLR side of the supine patient and if both sides are limited you stand at the side of greatest limitation.

We will firstly deal with the patient who has only a small loss or has a full but painful end range with SLR. You place his flexed knee over your shoulder as seen in Figure 29. You now ask him to push you away with his leg and then relax. At this point you push his bent knee up as far as you can in the direction of his shoulder on the same side provided there is no pain. If it is painful alter the direction by taking his leg more medially or laterally. Sustain this stretch for several seconds and then lower the leg to the bed. With the bent knee over your shoulder you include a traction component with this technique. When indicated the stretch does not hurt and after being repeated three times you expect a marked improvement when they again straight leg raise.

Let us now consider the patient with a gross loss of SLR. Maybe he can only SLR to 20 degrees. Place one hand under his knee and clasp under his heel with the other. You flex, and keep, his knee to 20 degrees and raise the heel just off the bed. The patient is now asked to push his leg down to the bed against your resistance and then relax. At this point you raise the leg gently as far as you can from the bed, maintaining the knee flexion and introducing some hip abduction at the same time. There must be no pain. If painful alter the direction of the raise medially or laterally. If still painful abandon the technique. As with the knee over your shoulder repeat three times and then reassess.

Figure 29

The bent leg raise technique.

After the successful application of a bent leg raise technique you can then carry out your other therapies. When a patient points out to you how much better he is after this therapy your only reply need be "Of course".

NB: A wonderful, yes wonderful, modification of the BLR procedure can be undertaken with the patient on his hands and knees. This can be done on the bed or floor. (See figure 30) The patient has his knees well apart. Keeping his hands in this starting position he flexes his knees and hips so that his "behind " moves towards the space provided between his feet. He "stretches out" his spine in this way , sustains the stretch then rocks forward for a rest and then repeats the stretch etc. Because his knees are apart, when viewed from the side the movement taking place is similar to that with the bent leg raise technique. Patients feel a grand sense of relief when doing this. They can sustain the stretch as long as they like and repeat many times and go through the sequence again and again during the day as they feel necessary provided they find that it is useful and of course with the technique they must experience no pain. If they did they would not use it. Even patients with an acute lesion will often find relief from it. Call it what you like but in our notes we record it as the "Lion Technique".

Figure 30
The "Lion Technique"

E. The two leg rotation technique also known as the "gate technique"

This is another superb procedure for lumbar spine lesions that restrict straight leg raising. To me it is special because when useful it can be done successfully by the patient without assistance. For many years I would apply the technique but now I teach my patients to do it so that between visits they can carry on the therapy. It is always combined with other routines of course. It would never be done if it caused pain and initially, until it is established that it is going to be useful, it is done slowly and gently and the "the rule of three" applies on the first visit.

Let us assume that our patient has limited straight leg raising on the right. He lies supine and grips the side of the plinth with his left hand. Both legs are now flexed so that the feet are off the plinth. Keeping his shoulders on the bed he takes his legs slowly to the side of the limited straight leg raise. (See figure 31a). He must feel no pain. If painful he alters the degree of flexion at the hips (more or less) to see if this enables further pelvic rotation. It usually will but he may again find further progress painful. If so again alter the degree of flexion at the hips and see if further progress may be made with the rotation. When he reaches his limit the position is sustained for several seconds before returning to a crook lying position. He then places first one leg then the other out straight on the bed. At this point SLR is measured. In nearly every case when the technique can be undertaken painlessly you will see an improvement. The whole process is repeated another two times when further progress will have been made. The patient is then instructed to repeat the treatment at regular intervals as you think fit.

This technique can be called the "gate technique" for the following reason. When the patient attempts to take his knees to the side of the limited straight leg raise the movement may stop as if he has encountered a barrier like a fence. By increasing or decreasing his hip flexion, further movement takes place as if he has found a gate in the fence and gone through it. He again may encounter a further barrier (fence) and with altered hip flexion finds the next "gate" to go through and so on. If he cannot find a "gate" then pain will warn you that the treatment is not appropriate.

Difficulties? There are two problems that you will encounter.

The first is apprehension. Some patients with very sore backs are very apprehensive of this technique. Let them measure and note their straight leg raise limitation and then coax them to gently try the technique but do not go too far. Return them to the starting position and let them remeasure their SLR. If it has visibly improved their attitude to the next rotation will be free from any apprehension.

The second is the bed on which they try to do their own two leg rotations. When using the plinth in your clinic they are normally able to rotate to a

Figure 31a

Two leg rotation technique for the lumbar spine. ("Gate" technique.)

position where their knees are over the side of the bed. This is not possible at home as the beds are too wide. What we suggest is that they place pillows under the hips which elevates them above the surface of the bed. The two leg rotation will now be more effective. (See figure 31b)

F. Straight leg raise with traction

The reason given in many texts as to why there is be pain (with or without limitation) on straight leg raising is because nerve tissue is being stretched over an obstruction. For the technique, about to be described , to work this theory cannot apply. However I will let you, the reader, be the judge of this. For this technique to work it is necessary that the patient can SLR to at least 40 degrees.

We have been able, using this technique, to improve the status of patients who have failed to respond to other therapies delivered by all sorts of manual therapy practitioners.

Figure 31b

Two leg rotation technique with pillows under hips to increase rotation.

Let us assume we have a patient who has right SLR loss which at the end of his available range produces a referred pain to his right posterior thigh. The patient is supine and you stand facing his right side. You get him to actively SLR without your assistance and you both note the range. You now grasp his lower leg proximal to the ankle joint and raise it off the bed to a position just short of the painful range. Flex your knees and hold the clasped leg to your chest. When you extend your knees this will effectively apply a longitudinal traction to the leg provided the bed is low enough and you are tall enough.(See figure 32) Sustain this traction and undertake a straight leg raise as far as it will go provided there is no pain. If there is pain you may find that it disappears if you slightly abduct or adduct the hip as you raise the leg. When pain free, SLR with traction three times and watch as the patient reassesses his SLR. There should be smiles all round.

When successful you may on subsequent visits do more than three repetitions and use over pressure provided there is no discomfort. To SLR with traction painlessly in this manner must surely defy the textbook rationale already mentioned.

Remember that the technique is only part of the therapy.

Figure 32
SLR with traction.

G. Spinal Mobilisations with Leg Movement. (SMWLM'S)

In section A of this book, sub-section 5, "Spinal Mobilisations with Arm Movement" were dealt with. Chronologically in my voyages of discovery in the field of manual therapy, spinal mobilisations with arm movement came first but it was not long before I discovered that by using the same principles the lumbar spine could also be treated when there was a loss of SLR or the patient presented with a positive Femoral Nerve Test. I consider this last technique to be the final chapter in the new field of MWM'S as they apply to the vertebral column. As time passes they will however been modified and improved upon. As a therapy they will earn an equal place with other manual therapies currently in use and when you read part two of this book you will be amazed at how extensively they can be applied in the treatment of extremity joints. Back to work!

Let us assume we have a patient with pain to the right knee when he straight leg raises to 45 degrees.

Have him facing you , lying on his left side. To undertake this technique you need an assistant. You flex over the patient and place one thumb reinforced by the other on the right side of Lumbar 4's spinous process. (See figure 33) This is often tender to touch so place a piece of plastic foam under your thumb. Now have your assistant abduct the patients leg passively approximately 10 degrees. They should support the leg by placing one hand under the ankle and the other under the knee. The knee should be very slightly bent.

Now push down on the chosen spinous process which will rotate that vertebra on the one below and at the same time have the patient actively SLR in the side lying position provided there is no pain. (See figure 34) As with the previous three techniques repeat three times then test again the straight leg raise when the patient is in a supine position. Satisfaction can almost be guaranteed but do no more than this on day one. On subsequent visits, as the patient improves, your assistant can apply overpressure, again with the understanding that there is no discomfort. Sometimes the spinous process to choose is lumbar 5 and when a patient has a positive femoral nerve sign lumbar 2 or 3 may be chosen. I hate to use superlatives, as the reader has probably already noticed, but when this technique works there is no other word for it other than exciting.

Figure 33

Spinal Mobilisations with Leg Movement. The thumbs push the chosen spinous process down to the bed effecting a rotation.

Figure 34

SMWLM's with assistant.

H. Sitting

One of the problems encountered when treating the lumbar spine is the difficulty that most patients have with sitting.

Kneeler chairs have proved useful but many cannot tolerate them because of knee complications and the fact that they have no back support. To place a lumbar roll assists in maintaining a lordosis but not a natural one when the hips are at 90 degrees to the trunk and the seat back is upright. We all know that when a patient sits the pressure within the lower lumbar disc is greater than when standing because of the pelvic tilt. The kneeler chair addresses this problem very nicely by lowering the knees and thus adjusting the pelvic tilt. We suggest that our patients sit on a simple stacking chair (see figure 35) with their legs apart so that they can lower their knees to lower the pressure on the bottom discs and thus form the natural lordosis they have when standing. As you will see from the photograph there is a convenient space for their "behinds" to fit in when they sit correctly right back in the chair and when positioned correctly the back pad gives appropriate support. The simple chair still posed a problem for ladies in particular as it is not an elegant sitting posture and some patients found that their hips were not flexible enough to straddle the chair. There was thus a need to modify the simple stacking chair to make it more acceptable. This was done by altering the pad that you sit on. (See figure 36a) This new chair is cheap to produce and is even useful for patients with say hip arthritis who have lost hip flexion and find a comfortable chair difficult to buy.

We have now made the chair a little more sophisticated by placing the basic design on wheels and a height adjustable stem. (See figure 36b).

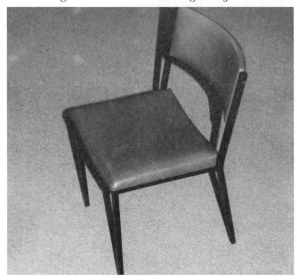

Figure 35

The simple stacking chair.

Figure 36a

The basic new chair design. Cheap and effective.

Figure 36b

The office chair.

F. Taping

I use rolls and rolls of 5 cm wide zinc oxide tape in my practice for I tape many spines.

As the upper thoracic spine is readily upset with poor posture and especially with over reaching, taping maintains a good posture and speeds up recovery. With some females I tie their brassiere straps at the back and this often assists.

Many patients experiencing pain with full end range neck rotation will be symptomless if you hold the shoulder girdle back when the movement takes place. If so tape them for a few days as in Figure 37.

With acute lower dorsal and lumbar lesions I tape the patient after "SNAGS" etc. This reminds them to maintain a good posture and they are grateful for this support. (See figure 37).

Figure 37

Transverse taping for the upper thoracic spine and cross taping for the lower thoracic or lumbar spines.

PART TWO

THE EXTREMITIES. MOBILISATIONS WITH MOVEMENT. (MWMs)

Explanation

There is nothing new in mobilisation and nothing new in movement to be dealt with in this section. It is the combination of the two modalities that is advocated. When successful the results that can be obtained are spectacular.

I consider them a breakthrough in the management of extremity joint restrictions and also in dealing with some apparent soft tissue lesions.

Mobilisations with movement (MWMs) will require professional validation to be included in the syllabi of orthodox manual therapy courses. However I predict that this will occur quickly once manipulative therapists become acquainted with and start to use them. To assist in their promotion I am building up a library of video material showing their efficacy on patients in my clinic. When I use these film clips on the lecture circuit they make a substantial impact on colleagues not to mention the patients involved at the time of their treatment.

The reader will observe that I did not specify active movement with mobilisation because there is a place for passive movement and certainly passive overpressure as well.

In addition there is a place for active contractions of muscles around a joint with mobilisation. The pain experienced with the standard muscle contraction tests for chronic "tennis elbow" will usually disappear when undertaken with an appropriate elbow joint mobilisation.

It would appear to me, the unscientific observer, that this new treatment approach (MWMs) is required for one basic reason.

I consider that minor positional faults occur following injury or strain resulting in movement restrictions and/or pain. These are not readily palpable or visible on x-ray but when a correctional mobilisation (a repositioning) is sustained, pain free function is restored and several repetitions will begin to bring lasting improvements. When the position of the ulna is altered with a sustained mobilisation in an elbow that has been restricted for many months and this enables the patient to immediately increase his range of movement this not only tells us something but is really exciting. I consider that this theory holds because when you just mobilise the joint in the same direction many times without the movement, and then check the active range there is no change.

Another reason that seems to confirm the position hypothesis is that the mobilisation with the movement is nearly always at right angles to the plane of the movement taking place and will only work in ONE direction. A further point is that when the correct MWM is repeated several times the joint's memory to stay on track seems to return.

These positional faults would appear to occur in all extremity joints and this possibility should be considered when assessing patients with joint problems. I have on film a young (14yrs) dancer who strained her foot and had been unable to plantar flex for three weeks because of pain. We found that a sustained mobilisation of the base of her second metatarsal down on the third enabled pain free plantar flexion. What was more remarkable was the fact that after several repetitions she was then able to plantar flex painlessly without the mobilisation (positional correction). Although some discomfort was present when she returned two days later further MWMs cleared this and she returned to dancing.

The reader will of course agree when comparing "SNAGS" with "MWMs" that there is very little difference. They both address the problems of movement pain and restriction, they both bring about a change at the time of delivery, they are painless when indicated and of course they are both examples of a sustained mobilisation with movement. The main difference between the spinal techniques and those for the extremities is that with the former the facet mobilisations are normally in the direction of the active movement taking place and with the extremities the sustained mobilisations to correct a positional fault are applied in a different direction to the movement glide taking place.

With many joints the correction can be maintained with taping. This new form of assessment and therapy began for me with a finger but we can now apply it, when indicated, to all peripheral joints.

Descriptions

Examples of how you may apply MWMs to different extremity joints will now be detailed. Sufficient examples will be given to enable the professional to fully understand the principles so that they will quickly be able to ascertain when, how and why they will use them.

1. The fingers. Loss of and/or pain with interphalangeal joint movement.

We all see patients with restricted hinge joint movement following injury and the fingers are no exception. A typical therapy routine would be some form of heat followed by active exercises and of course manual therapy. The manual therapy used by most would include traction, ventral or dorsal glides and maybe medial or lateral glides. In my decades as a therapist I have rarely been able to achieve instant success with this format. MWMs are so good as a treatment modality with restricted finger movement that I would humbly suggest they should be your first choice of therapy. I extol their supremacy for two reasons. Firstly the glides are painless as is the active movement taking place. Secondly the restricted range of movement is immediately altered. It is paramount to remember that this therapy should be painless and if not discard it. Another point is that if the range of movement does not alter straight away discard the technique. Simple!

The patient is seated and you stabilise the proximal facet of the stiff and often swollen joint with the pads of your right (or left) index finger and thumb. These are placed medially and laterally. Now secure the distal facet of the joint medially and laterally with your other thumb and index finger. (See figure 38). The distal facet is now glided medially and then laterally. In nearly every case you will find that one direction is painful and the other is not. You choose the direction that is painless and then ask the patient to flex his stiff finger while you sustain the mobilisation. This active movement should be pain free and the range should increase. To improve the MWM have the patient apply some overpressure with his free hand. This overpressure is like the cream on the milk. It enhances the result. This procedure would be repeated several times and the range of movement reassessed.

When we talk about a medial or lateral glide it should be added that the application requires some sensitivity. Remember it must be parallel with the treatment plane. A pain being experienced with a particular glide will often disappear by minimally altering the direction. When you get an instant improvement in a range of movement with a sustained glide in one direction only, which is at right angles to the glide taking place, what other explanation could there be for its success other than the correction of a positional fault?

In the past five years I have had four patients who have not responded to a medial or lateral glide with movement but to a rotation of the distal facet with movement. The first patient was memorable. She was unable to flex the metacarpo/phalangeal of her thumb following a hyperextension injury. Full of confidence I said to her that she would be able to move the joint immediately and without pain when I placed the bone ends in the correct position. To my surprise and well hidden embarrassment I found that neither a medial or a lateral glide made any difference. However because of my conversion to the positional fault belief I tried a medial rotation of the distal facet on the proximal but this was painful. I then rotated the facet in the opposite direction. Brilliant! No pain and she was able to again move her joint. The other three who failed to respond to the glide at right angles also responded to the appropriate rotation. (Aristotle said that you can trust your judgement if it is based on logic?)

When teaching I now tell participants that with mobile hinge joints, excluding the ankle, the appropriate mobilisation to use with movement is usually at right angles to the glide taking place and if these are painful try a rotation.

With fingers the technique is so simple that patients can be taught to do their own MWMs several times a day. As already mentioned you can expect, when these techniques are indicated and applied, to find that the patient has retained most of the improvement gained at his next treatment session.

2. The metacarpals. Pain when the hand is clenched along say the 5th metacarpal.

There are no joints between adjacent metacarpals. However be on the alert for postitional faults between all adjacent long bones in the body. An excellent example that I must share with you was of a women who three months after a fracture of her fifth metacarpal had pain whenever she gripped anything. The pain was over the proximal third of the bone and she experienced a lot of pain gripping the steering wheel of her car. We found that when the base of the fifth metacarpal was lifted up in relation to the fourth her grip was pain free. Three sets of these MWM'S resulted in pain free gripping without the correction.

She returned two days later feeling much better and only required four

Figure 38

MWM for loss of interphalangeal joint flexion or extension.

treatments. I should add that I taped the base of the fifth metacarpal up on the fourth before she left my rooms to ensure that the bone remained in "the corrected position".

3. The carpal bones

Mobilisations with movement have proved to be the solution with many patients with localised functional pain in the carpus. An example would be a patient who experiences pain over the dorsal aspect of his Trapezium with gripping. In my teaching video a patient is presented with such a problem of 9 months' duration and followed a crush injury. Specialists were unable to offer an explanation for his misery. We found that by "repositioning " his trapezius ventrally in relation to the scaphoid he could clench his fist with no discomfort. I must admit that it took several attempts to get the right direction of the glide so that there was no discomfort. As with the earlier MWMs we would have him gripping strongly 10 times with the sustained mobilisation. After three sets he would depart almost pain free and after six treatments was discharged.

On my courses I now teach that with joints in the body that only have small ranges of movement, the mobilisation with movement is really to reposition one facet up or down on its neighbour with movement as an assessment to see if it is indicated. The other point that I make after dealing with the fingers, metacarpals and carpus, is that on the basis of the MWMs for these joints you now have guidelines to assess and treat when indicated all the joints of the body.

As you read on you will see how pertinent these comments are.

4. The wrist joint. A loss of and pain with flexion and/or extension.

As with the fingers the accompanying mobilisation with the movement is usually a medial or lateral glide. I have found that in every case the successful glide has been a lateral one and I would like to describe this first of all.

The patient is seated. You stand proximal to and grasp the lower ends of the radius and ulna with one hand so that the web between your index finger and thumb lies over the distal end of the radius. The web between the thumb and index finger of your other hand lies medially over the proximal row of carpal bones keeping the rest of your finger and thumb from making contact with the patient. (See figure 39). You now glide the carpals laterally and while maintaining the mobilisation have the patient actively move in the restricted direction. (Flexion or extension). If the MWM is indicated the range of movement will improve instantly and of course painlessly. Repeat ten times having the patient apply overpressure with his free hand to get further range. After three sets of ten the patient should now find that they can move, without positional correction, much more freely.

A useful adjunct to a successful MWM is to apply tape diagonally across the wrist joint to maintain the useful glide.(See figure 40).

It may interest the reader to know that we recently treated a 35 year old woman who presented with a dorsal wrist ganglion as well as pain and a loss of wrist flexion. The ganglion and painful movement loss followed a jarring injury three weeks earlier. With our first sustained lateral glide she was able to fully flex her wrist painlessly and the ganglion immediately reduced in size. After six repetitions she had full pain free function and the swelling had dissipated. We were fortunate enough to record her treatment at the time on video tape.

If a lateral glide is not successful in allowing pain free movement you rotate the proximal row of carpals on the radius and ulna to see if this repositioning allows the wrist to function. As to whether you rotate medially or laterally is for you to find out. The reader will now see that the approach is no different to that taken with a finger. The rotation can be sustained with taping and we found this taping extremely effective in removing pain and swelling from the osteoarthritic wrist of a 65 year old woman.

Figure 39

MWM for wrist joint flexion or extension

Figure 40

Taping to maintain lateral glide of carpals at the wrist.

5. The distal Radio ulnar joint. Pain and/or movement loss with pronation or perhaps supination.

With this joint an altered relationship between the distal ends of the radius an ulna can cause pain and movement loss. To check if this is the case grasp the lower end of the radius between the thumb and index finger of one hand and the lower end of the ulna with your other hand. (See figure 41). First glide the ulna ventrally on the radius and have the patient actively move in the painful direction. (Pronation or supination). If this is painful, glide the ulna dorsally with the offending movement. If the MWM is indicated then no pain will be experienced with movement and several repetitions will make a tremendous difference. It would then be easy to tape the ulna in its corrected position if you thought it desirable. For this technique to work I assume that there is a positional fault and using this technique on one of my courses in America a therapist with a 12 year loss of pronation regained her full movement in one session before 30 colleagues. It made quite an impact.

Figure 41

MWM for forearm supination or pronation loss with pain at distal radio-ulnar joint.

6. The elbow joint. Movement losses and Tennis Elbow.

Basically the elbow is a hinge joint and this prompted me to experiment with the above conditions to see if MWMs might apply in their treatment and they most certainly do. In 1990 I succeeded in dramatically improving an 8 year loss of flexion in a 44 year old man in one treatment session. This was certainly exceptional and I have video corroboration of this.

a. Movement losses.

The patient is lying on his back with his arm on the plinth and forearm supinated. You wrap the now familiar belt around your hips and his forearm so that the proximal edge is level with the elbow joint. You stabilise the lower end of his humerus with one hand and support the forearm with the other. (See figure 42a). You now glide the ulna laterally with the belt by moving you hips gently away. Little force is used. Provided there is no pain the patient then actively bends or extends his elbow while you maintain the mobilisation. You can add a little overpressure with your distally placed hand. If the patient is extending, remember that with the carrying angle at the elbow, the treatment plane alters slightly with the movement and you must alter the direction of your glide to deal with this. Depending on your size and that of the patient's elbow you may choose not to use a belt. Instead you can secure the lower end of the humerus with one hand and apply the glide with your other hand. To do this position the lateral border of the 2nd metacarpal of your free hand over the upper end of the ulna at the joint margin. (See figure 42b).

The reader will note from the photograph that I make no skin contact with the rest of my mobilising hand. I do not want it to block movement. When both hands are busy in this way I get the patient to apply passive overpressure to the movement.

As with all the other mobilisations already dealt with in this book remember that other forms of therapy would be given as well.

b. Tennis elbow.

With long standing tennis elbows we have been using a new routine involving MWMs and have had some interesting successes.

The treatment is to make the patient exercise his forearm repeatedly in any way that is (on testing) painful but . . . the exercise is done with a sustained mobilisation and must be painless. (See figure 43). Let us assume that the patient is unable, when the elbow is extended and the

Figure 42a

MWM for elbow movement loss. Lateral glide with belt.

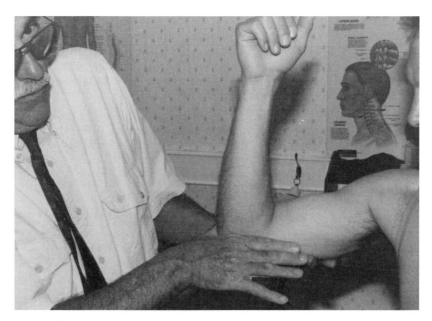

Figure 42b

MWM for elbow movement loss using hands.

forearm pronated, to clench his fist without pain. We have found that in nearly every case when a lateral glide is applied at the elbow joint the patient experiences no pain. When this has been repeated many times he is then able to clench the fist without discomfort and without the concurrent mobilisation. Interesting? Be it painful wrist or finger extension or gripping pain the same lateral glide seems to work. Sometimes it takes three or four attempts to get the gliding direction exactly right but when on target it's great. We usually, as an assessment, use our hands rather than the belt to ascertain the efficacy of the technique as described for elbow restrictions. (See figure 42b). For these MWMs to work with what is thought to be a soft tissue lesion there must be a tracking or positional fault at the elbow contributing in no small way to the tennis elbow.

We still use tennis elbow bracing and other therapy at the same time. The patients are instructed to exercise regularly at home. They are shown how to self mobilise so that the exercises are pain free. If they cannot successfully self mobilise then the exercises are not given.

One way of self gliding the extended elbow is to use a doorway. Stand with the upper arm against the wall so that the elbow joint is level with the opening. Now push the ulna laterally using the web space between the index finger and thumb of the free hand. (See figure 43a). After a few sets of self MWMs the patient should be able to exercise without pain.

Sometimes with tennis elbow the grip is painful through a range of elbow flexion so the MWMs would be undertaken with altered elbow flexion. A variation to the lateral glide with movement has been required with some tennis elbows when pain has been produced with gripping when the elbow was at a right angle. When the flexed elbow was distracted with a belt the pain with gripping was eliminated. (See figure 43b).

While on the subject of Tennis Elbow could I refer the reader back to the section on Cervical Mobilisations with Arm Movements. If MWMs do not work or there are still a residual symptoms after their use try moving Cervical 4 (or 5) across away from the affected side and re test for tennis elbow. Worth a try and I will say no more.

7. The shoulder joint. Painful movement losses, rotator cuff lesions etc.

The applications of MWMs for shoulder joint lesions can be rewarding. They certainly have a place and in this new edition I wish to deal with some of the uses for them. Historically my first "miracle" using MWMs on a shoulder occurred in 1990. A 28 year old lass on treatment for her neck had been unable to raise her arm actively from her side more than 20 degrees, in any direction, for 10 years. She had always had a full passive range of movement and there was no obvious explanation for the prob-

Figure 43

MWM for tennis elbow using belt in lying.

Figure 43a

Self MWM for tennis elbow using doorway.

Figure 43b

MWM. Distraction with movement at elbow using belt.

lem. She naturally had weakness from disuse but none of the specialists she had consulted had ever been able to give any reason for the movement loss. Shortly before the symptoms appeared she strained her shoulder tramping. From the time of her first visit, when MWMs were used, she was able to abduct to 90 degrees and after that treatment steadily improved. She followed a supervised program of self MWMs and over three months made a full recovery.

Let us consider the application of MWMs to a right shoulder that is painful when raised above 90 degrees through abduction (typical with a rotator cuff lesion). The patient is seated. You stand at his left side with your right hand over his left scapula and the thenar eminence of your left hand over the head of the humerus. You ask the patient to raise his arm up from his side while you apply a posterior gliding force over the head of the humerus with your left hand. (Avoid pressure over the sensitive corocoid process). (See figure 44) When indicated and you are correctly positioned the arm will rise painlessly. As with the finger, wrist and elbow, the mobilisation that seems to work is at right angles to the active glide taking place. Is it a positional fault that inhibits pain free movement? If the technique is successful the next step is to have the patient repeat the movement under load by giving them a weight to lift as in the Figure 44. You will note that I said to push the head of the humerus posteriorly. We have never had any success with an anterior glide but this possibility should not be excluded. As with the MWMs for the other joints, after several repetitions, patients should notice a marked improvement and much of this should be retained between visits. Many quickly learn how to apply their own MWMs. This technique has proved instantly successful with

Figure 44
MWM for shoulder elevation through abduction

some patients who have a gross loss of movement, usually with some swelling, following a fall on or a blow to their shoulder.

To dorsally glide the humerus of a large patient, when you are small in stature, is simple when you use a belt. (See figure 45) You stand behind the seated patient and place the belt around both your hips and the patient's shoulder. Place a hand on the scapular for fixation and lean back in such a way as to glide the humeral head back in the treatment plane. Ensure that the belt does not slightly elevate the humeral head as this will jam the joint and inhibit movement. Remember no pain and the usual repetitions etc.

Another movement loss that can respond spectacularly to a MWM is internal rotation provided the patient can get his thumb around as far as his sacrum. (See figure 46a).

For a loss of right internal rotation stand facing the patient's right side. Place your right thumb in the bend of his flexed right elbow. His hand should be as far behind his back as possible. Now place the web between your finger and thumb in the patient's axilla. You now glide the head of the humerus down in the glenoid fossa using your thumb while stabilising the scapula with your left hand. Make sure the your left hand is stabilising up and inwards. If not you will place a pressure on the upper end of the humerus which is both unpleasant and ineffective. While this distrac-

Figure 45

MWM with abduction using belt.

Figure 46a

MWM for internal rotation.

Figure 46b

MWM for internal rotation using belt.

Manual Therapy

tion is taking place have the patient internally rotate his shoulder, with the help of the other hand if necessary, while you adduct his upper arm with your abdomen. As you push into adduction in this way the head of the humerus is distracted laterally. The hand in the axilla acts as a fulcrum. It all sounds very complex but it is not difficult to do and patients amazingly tolerate the technique and experience no pain. What is more important is that in most cases internal rotation is increased.

There is an alternative way of doing this using your treatment belt instead of your thumb.(See figure 46a) Place the belt in the bend of the elbow and have the loop about 6 centimetres from the floor when it lies obliquely behind the patient's back. For the right shoulder place your left forefoot in the loop ensuring that your heel is on the floor. As the belt lies obliquely, when pressure is applied in the bend of the elbow as your foot plantarflexes, the emphasis is where your thumb would have been. That is right on the joint margin which does not prevent the forearm from flexing up behind the back. Your two overlapping hands are placed in the axilla to stabilise the scapula and they thus act as a greater fulcrum when you use your abdomen to adduct the arm behind the patient's back.

8. The foot

Foot injuries abound due to the participation in impact sporting activities by an increasing percentage of the public at large over recent years. Never before have the streets of our cities been so overwhelmed with runners and there has been a proliferation of fitness centres crammed with devotees.

To introduce you to the application of mobilisations with movement as a foot therapy I will deal with two areas where pain with movement can be experienced. However when foot movement causes localised foot pain a "MWM" should always be tried. It can quickly be established if it is indicated as it would allow the offending movement to take place painlessly.

a. Pain over the medial border of the foot with inversion.

This can be due to a "positional" fault at the base of the first metatarsal. The patient's foot is on a plinth. You stand beside and proximal to the foot to be treated. (Let us assume a left one). You place the ventral shaft of the first metacarpal of your right hand along the dorsum of the shaft of the patient's first metatarsal. The fingers of this hand lie firmly beneath this metatarsal so the bone is secured. The fingers of your left hand lie under the foot along the shaft of the second metatarsal.(See figure 47). Now glide the base of the first metatarsal down on the second and while maintaining this ask the patient to invert the foot provided there is no pain. Your fingers beneath the second metetarsal apply a counter pressure up on the second metatarsal. If the inversion is now pain free have the patient repeat the movement with mobilisation many times. (Ten?). When successful they will now have painless active inversion without mobilisation. To assist your therapy a positional taping can be used for a few days.

Although it is usually a ventral glide that works it may be the other direction that is required so you alter your hand placements for the MWMs.

b. Anterior metatarsalgia. Pain under the transverse arch.

If pain under the heads of the middle metatarsals can be reproduced with toe flexion or extension this could be due to a metatarsal head positional fault and a MWM should be tried.

With the patient's foot on the plinth stand proximal and grasp the head of say the third metatarsal between the soft pads of your thumb and index finger. Your other thumb and index finger grasps the head of the adjacent second. Now glide and hold the third down on the second while the patient flexes his toes. (See figure 48). If painful, glide the second down on the third.

When painless repeat six to ten times and then have the patient flex his toes without assistance to reassess. After several sets he should feel much better. We would follow this therapy with corrective exercises and perhaps appropriate taping.

Figure 47

MWM for pain with inversion along medial border of foot.

Figure 48

Metatarsalgia. MWM. Technique for patient experiencing pain with toe flexion or extension.

9. The Ankle Joint

The ankle joint is a delight to treat when there is a loss of plantar or dorsiflexion and the technique I will describe for the former I call the 100% miracle technique and the techniques for dorsiflexion I call the 97% miracle techniques. Both of course are MWMs but the former was in fact shown to me by Professor F M Kaltenborn in 1974. It was not taught as an MWM of course and sadly the significance of the procedure escaped me (and others) for many years.

a. Plantar flexion loss.

Let us assume that your patient has a loss of movement in his right ankle. He reclines on a couch with his right knee flexed and heel on the bed and you stand at the end facing him. Place the hypothenar border of your right hand just proximal to the joint line and wrap your thumb and fingers around the lower leg. (See figure 49)

Now place the webbing between the thumb and index finger of your left hand around the talus. Your thumb and index fingers would slope slightly distally so that they lie just below the malleolae. Stand in a lunge position with your right elbow wedged in your right groin. Using your body weight

Figure 49
"Miracle" MWM for ankle plantar flexion.

glide the tibia and fibula posteriorly as far as you can. This locks the ankle joint. Without releasing this glide roll the talus ventrally with your left hand. Very little movement is expected due to the slack being taken up in the joint by your right arm. What movement you do get is in fact restored plantar flexion. Several repetitions ensure a marked and lasting improvement.

Patients would exercise to maintain the range.

Forgive the tedious reminders but this MWM must not hurt. Often after fractures the tissues around the ankle are swollen and thus tender. As on other occasions use some plastic foam under your hands for patient comfort.

b. Dorsiflexion loss.

Let us assume that your patient has a loss of movement in his right ankle.

The patient lies on the treatment table with his ankle joint level with the end of the bed. Under his tendo achilles place a small pad to fill the space. Grasp the calcaneum securely with your left hand and wrap your right hand over the front of the foot so that it lies over the talus. Then pull the calcaneum down towards the floor with your left hand while at the same time gliding the talus down with your right hand. To do this just slightly bend your knees which makes the manoeuvre effortless. Sustain this glide and ask the patient to actively dorsiflex. When they respond the tendons over the ventral ankle joint force your right hand from the talus so you relax and then ask the patient to relax. When they stop dorsiflexing use you lower abdomen to retain the movement by leaning forward. Your left hand does not relax and continues to sustain the glide of the calcaneum and with it the talus posteriorly. You repeat the glide down with your right hand and again ask the patient to further dorsi flex and so on . . .

Another way to do this is with the patient standing on a bed with the restricted ankle in front, and thus weightbearing. Place the ever useful belt around your hips and the patient's lower leg. Between the belt and the tendo achilles you must place a thick piece of plastic foam. (See figure 51) Now wrap the web between the thumb and index finger of one hand, reinforced by the other around the talus as close to the joint margin as possible. The belt gives fixation to the tibia and fibula while you glide the talus dorsally. At the same time the patient actively forces further dosiflexion by flexing his knee. For safety an extra person could hold his hand. (How nice!) Several repetitions please and reassess.

Figure 50

97% "Miracle" MWM for ankle dorsi flexion.

Figure 51
Weightbearing MWM for ankle dorsi flexion.

10. The tibio/fibular joints.

a. The distal tibio/fibular joint.

In dealing with this joint I would like to suggest that all practitioners in the medical and allied medical fields have been so so wrong in the diagnosis of many ankle strains. I believe and also hope to convince you that a large percentage of patients diagnosed as having strained the lateral ligament of the ankle have not. The problem resulting from inversion strains lies within the distal tibio/fibular joint. I believe that when the foot is inverted beyond the expected range the lateral ligament often remains virtually undamaged. The fibula gets wrenched forward on the tibia and positional faults occur.

To describe the technique let me do so with a case history. In 1992 a middle aged man limped in to see me 6 weeks after he "went over" on his ankle. His foot was swollen and he had no inversion at all. On assessment I found that when I glided his fibula back on his tibia and held it there he was able to fully invert his foot with NO PAIN. After the usual MWM repetitions I taped his fibula dorsally on his tibia and he left my rooms feeling 90% better. On his return two days later most of his swelling had gone and he had only minimal discomfort at the end of full range inversion. MWMs were again used and no further therapy was required. A gratifying result and to me the only explanation that my simple mind can accept is that he had a positional fault. Ever since, with all "lateral ligament" strains of the ankle we have checked the fibula and I am confident that ankle strains rarely damage the lateral ligament. Most strains involve the tibio/fibular "joint". Referring back to the man above I wish to make the following points. Firstly after 6 weeks if the only damage to his ankle was to the lateral ligament why had it not shown any signs of recovery. The swelling could be explained but not the gross loss of inversion. Secondly when the foot is inverted while you are gliding the fibula dorsally the stretch on the lateral ligament is increased. Why did he feel no pain and why was he now able to fully invert his foot? My explanation, and it is hard to refute it, is that gliding the fibula on the tibia returned the bone to its correct position allowing pain free function to occur. In England last year (1994) a therapist on one of my courses had ankle pains and had been unable to invert her foot for 13 years. The fibula was glided dorsally and while the position was maintained she was able to get a full active range of inversion. Course participants almost in unison when they saw this mini "miracle" said "what about adaptive shortening?" I did not answer their question but the result would have left a lasting impact on all of them. (It was suggested that I might like to go for a walk on the Lake afterwards). (Study figure 52).

Figure 52
The distal tibio-fibular joint MWM for inversion.

When you glide the fibula down and pain is experienced, just minimally alter the direction of the movement. You might not have the treatment plane direction right. We have also repositioned the fibula dorsally with tape to see if this assists in the management of "shin splints" and at times have been rewarded.

The MWM for a loss of eversion with or without pain is to try positioning the fibula ventrally on the tibia while the patient is in prone lying.

Remember overpressure should be used.

Figure 53

The proximal tibio-fibular joint MWM with weightbearing knee flexion.

b. The proximal tibio/fibular joint.

Be on the lookout for "positional faults" when postero/lateral knee pain is being experienced. Take for example the patient who experiences pain in this area with weightbearing knee flexion. Have your patient do this while you are gliding the fibular head forward on the tibia. A good way to achieve this is to have the patient place his foot on a chair and then flex forward over it. (see figure 53). If pain free, do three sets of ten MWMs and reassess. When successful the patient may be able to bend over and SELF MWM. Taping is extremely useful for keeping the fibula head "in position".

Patients with the remnants of sciatica down the lateral border of the lower leg to the foot will often experience no pain when the fibula is positioned in this way. This may be because it alters the tension on the nerve responsible.

You will note that my descriptions for MWMs are becoming briefer but it would be tedious to the reader if this were not so. Getting to this stage in the book and with the guidelines mentioned for the fingers, metacarpals and carpus earlier in this section you will probably be orchestrating your own MWMs as different joints are dealt with. This was how I have had to work my way through the joints.

12. The knee joint

As with the elbow, MWMs should always be tried when there is a loss of movement that is obviously not the result of serious trauma. The general rule for the gliding direction that I use with movement is "medial glide with medial knee pain and lateral glide with lateral knee pain". MWMs are much more likely to assist with a flexion loss than extension. This loss is usually the result of a sporting injury and is often seen when the patient is referred with a diagnosis of collateral ligament strain.

The patient lies prone and to apply a medial glide you stand on the contralateral side. Place a belt around your waist and the patient's lower leg so that the proximal edge is at the tibial joint margin. To do this you would of course expect the patient to have a reasonable degree of knee flexion. You stabilise the thigh above the knee with one hand and support the lower leg with the other. (See figure 54a). You glide the knee medially with the belt and ask the patient to flex his knee. When indicated the range of movement will immediately improve painlessly. To apply a lateral glide stand beside the restricted knee and use the belt to apply the glide as you did from the other side.

Alternative technique

I have already generalised in stating that with hinge joints the mobilisation used with movement is usually a medial or lateral glide. However in young adults, particularly sports' persons, who have lost full flexion after leg injuries requiring prolonged immobilisation there is another MWM that can be extremely useful. With this technique the tibial plateau is glided posteriorly (N.B. the treatment plane) first and then the patient flexes his knee while the glide is sustained. It is necessary to have at least 80 degrees of flexion before this procedure can be tried.

The patient is supine and you stand beside the knee to be treated. Interlace the fingers of both hands and place them over the flexed knee so that the heel of one hand lies over the tibial plateau, and the heel of the other is over the lower end of the femur. (See figure 54b). You can now successfully glide the upper end of the tibia posteriorly when you try to proximate the heels of your hands. It is amazing how powerful this technique is so take some care. If you are not right on the joint or your direction is slightly out it can be very painful. The patient's contribution here is very important. We usually attach a belt to the ankle of the patient on the restricted side and have her hold this with her hands. When you glide the tibia the patient then actively tries to flex her knee and gets some overpressure by cautiously pulling on the belt. The new position is held for a few seconds and after a short spell the MWM is repeated several times. When indicated the range should increase with each MWM even though it is only a few degrees. It should produce strain and discomfort but not pain. Strong young adults are ideal subjects for this technique but I would not use it on older or younger patients because of the force that can be applied so effortlessly.

Figure 54a

MWM. Medial glide with active knee flexion.

Figure 54b

MWM. Dorsal glide with active knee flexion.

13. The hip joint

As with other mobile joints, where possible the glide with movement should be at right angles to the movement glide. (i.e. Medial or lateral glide with finger flexion). I will only detail two useful MWMs and leave the rest for the reader as a professional to sort out.

a. Loss of internal rotation.

One of the movement losses that inculpates the hip joint is internal rotation, and provided the patient does not have too much joint deterioration on X-ray this mobilisation is excellent even if I say so myself. Let us assume that your patient has a loss of medial rotation in her right hip.

She lies on a treatment couch with her hip and knee flexed. Your treatment belt is around her upper thigh and around your upper thighs just below your hip joints. It is essential that the belt is as high as it will go on the patient otherwise the belt will be painful and the glide ineffective. Your bent left elbow is now placed in your left groin and the hand is placed on her lateral ilium. The forearm is inside the belt. When in position the belt must have no slack. (See figure 55). Wrap your right arm around the patient's thigh and lower leg. This is positioned so that you will be able to passively internally rotate the hip while you laterally glide the femur using your thighs to do this via the belt. Your left forearm, positioned as it is, stabilises the pelvis and is the key to the success of the treatment. Using this technique will in nearly every case painlessly improve the range of rotation thus improving the patient's function and reducing the pain. Sets of these are done and the patient is encouraged to do appropriate exercises at home.

b. To restore hip flexion

The technique is exactly the same as for rotation. Instead of passively rotating the hip you passively flex it with you free hand while the glide is applied laterally.

Figure 55

MWM. For hip rotation.

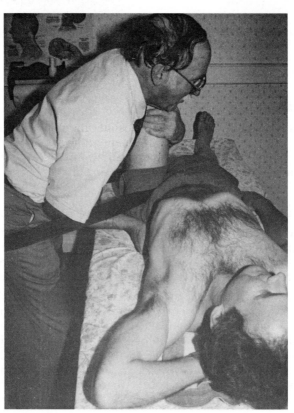

Final comments on mobilisations with movement

Remember with all applications of MWMs for painful joint restrictions, that the direction of your glide is critical. Pain may be produced if you are slightly off the treatment plane. Minor alterations to the gliding direction can make a tremendous difference.

Remember that MWMs when indicated are never painful.

Remember to do a sufficient number of repetitions as by doing so they have a more lasting effect and seem to jog the memory of the joint to stay on track or in position.

Remember to instruct the patients whenever possible to do their own MWMs.

Remember whenever possible to tape the patient's joint in a corrected position for a few days.

Remember that other forms of therapy can be given concurrently.

Remember to use them as part of your assessment to see if they are indicated.

Finally . . . Remember to use them even if they are revenue reducing.

PART THREE

THE EXTREMITIES. A POT POURRI.

Introduction

The reader will find this an unusual title for a treatise on the extremities but I wish to deal with some innovations for old techniques plus some old and new ideas of my own that I am sure physiotherapists will find of value.

My interest in manual therapy for the extremities was fired after attending my first course on this subject in 1970. It was in Helsinki and conducted by my early mentor Freddy Kaltenborn. I have of course been influenced, extremity wise, by the teachings of G Maitland whose name is synonymous with manual therapy and many others including J Cyriax, R Elvey, J Mennell and J McConnell.

I will at first discuss compression as a treatment then write about a new concept which I call the Pain Release Phenomenon ("PRP") to which compression therapy relates. "PRP"s have a wide application. They are still being developed and the reader who understands what I am on about will be able to apply "PRP"s in the treatment of many chronic conditions. This section will conclude with other useful extremity techniques.

A. COMPRESSION TREATMENTS FOR EXTREMITY JOINTS

Preamble

I started using compression in treatment regimes soon after reading the excellent article of G D Maitland's, "The Hypothesis of Adding Compression When Examining and Treating Synovial Joints" (6) in 1981. Although a very useful tool in manual therapy it soon became apparent that if safe guidelines were not developed and understood then some patients would have their conditions exacerbated and others denied this form of therapy. I would like to elaborate on the guidelines I use and then refer to some specific applications.

1. COMPRESSION AS A TEST

Description

As stated in Maitland's article, when assessing extremity joints you should try a compression test to see if this produces pain. To do this the joint is placed in a biomechanical resting position where all the structures surrounding it are maximally relaxed. You now stabilise the proximal facet with one hand and apply a compressive force on the joint with the other. While maintaining this compression try a series of joint movements to see if they produce pain. The movements to the joint would be those used in passive testing (e.g. flexion, extension, rotation etc.) or accessory movements (glides).

When using these tests avoid end range movement. You are looking for articular pain and if the joint is moved to end range then pain experienced may be capsular or ligamentous. Common sense must prevail re the amount of compression used. Excessive force is not needed and if the bone ends are painful it will cause unnecessary distress.

2. COMPRESSION AS A TREATMENT

Description

As already stated compression treatments come under the heading I call the "Pain Release Phenomenon" or conveniently "PRP". I will deal with "PRP"s in detail later in this section but at this point suffice to say that 20 seconds seems to be a "magical" time for compression as a treatment and other "PRP" treatments. Let me explain further.

If a combination of compression and movement causes pain then repeat the combination for up to 20 seconds to see if the pain disappears. Ensure that the pressure on the articular surfaces remains constant. If the pain increases then STOP immediately. Use no more pressure than that required to just produce the pain. If too much is used then that may be why the pain increases. I cannot over emphasize the importance of using the correct amount of compression. If the pain disappears within 20 seconds then a compression treatment is indicated. This means that you repeat the movement with the same amount of compression. The pain will go again within 20 seconds. Further repetitions see a remarkable change in the response of the joint surfaces. After several repetitions the time for the pain to go drops rapidly. Soon there is virtually no pain with the movement and this should signal the end of the first treatment session. On subsequent visits other movements producing pain with compression would be tried. It may become necessary to apply compression at end range. By this time if the pain goes you know it was still articular. If it does not it would indicate the source of pain is elsewhere. As therapists become skilled in using compression they will find them more useful than originally thought.

I mentioned that if the pain increased with movement and compression you would stop but if the pain does not abate after 20 seconds can I reiterate that it may be because too much force was used. Try it again with less compression and see what happens.

This 20 second guideline will ensure that no patients are ever exacerbated. The exception to this time span has been the patella. We have found that with some chronic knees 25 seconds would be acceptable. In countries where patients are quick to take action against a therapist if they feel worse these rules will be welcome.

Some compression applications worth mentioning

N.B. Although I will only mention certain joints remember it is a valid treatment option for any synovial joint where compression pain can be produced.

(1). The metatarso-phalangeal joint of the second toe or perhaps the third or fourth.

Patients often present with pain over the heads of their metatarsals. It may be diagnosed as metatarsalgia. A compression test is always warranted and if positive then a compression treatment is given. You often get a spectacular result relieving the patient after some months of misery. To do this the patient is lying. You grasp the base of the proximal phalanx of the second toe between your right (or left) thumb and first phalanx of your flexed index finger. The thumb and index finger of your other hand secures the head of the second metatarsal. (See figure 56). The base of the first phalanx is now glided up and down on the head of the second metatarsal while a moderate compression force is sustained. Try not to pinch when gripping and ensure your glide is a pure one with no wedging. The direction of the glide is oblique and when parallel with the treatment plane the range of movement is unexpectedly considerable when considering the size of the bone ends. If pain is experienced then compress with the glide for up to 20 seconds. If the pain goes within this time span repeat the procedure several times until a satisfactory result is obtained. Remember not to over compress and if the pain increases then stop immediately. As with all the other techniques dealt with in this book other treatments would still be given such as lumbrical exercises etc.

(2). The sesamoids beneath the first metatarso-phalangeal joint

The sesamoids can be suspected of causing weightbearing pain under the base of the big toe when the metatarso- phalangeal joint itself appears on examination to be symptomless.

Compression testing is a valid way of inculpating the wee bones as the cause of pain in their vicinity, under the medial border of the foot. As they are not easy to palpate I use the following routine to test them. Place the lateral border of the fully flexed index finger beneath the sesamoids and opposing thumb on top of the first metatarso-phalangeal joint. Us-

Figure 56

Compression treatment to the second metatarso-phalangeal joint.

Figure 57

Compression treatment for the sesamoids.

ing the flexed index finger provides a larger surface to place under these small bones and ensures they do not escape the compression about to be applied. (See figure 57). By squeezing with the thumb and index finger so positioned, the sesamoids cannot avoid the compression.

You now passively flex and extend the big toe. If pain is produced with this movement then it is probably coming from the sesamoids, particularly if it stops when the compression component is removed. Care must be taken not to compress the tendon of extensor longus hallicus on the bones beneath as it can be very tender. By off centring the pad of the thumb on top this can be avoided. If compression is painful then use it as a treatment following the 20 second rule. Only a few treatments are usually required. I must mention that I give exercises to strengthen the flexor longus hallicus muscle which is invariably weak and I use 2.5 cm wide zinc oxide strapping to reposition the sesamoids. The latter is done because the sesamoids in the foot are similar to the patella and pathologies can be managed in a similar way. Here I must refer the reader to Jenny McConnell's article "The Management of Chondromalacia Patellar - A Long Term Solution". (7). Her contribution in this field has been immense. The adhesive tape is attached to the sesamoids via the skin which enables them to be pulled medially. To maintain this new position the other end of the tape is wrapped over the dorsum of the foot.

(3). The metatarso-cuboid joint

In my experience I have yet to encounter a restriction between the 4th and 5th metatarsals and the cuboid. However in patients presenting with pain in this joint's vicinity especially on weight bearing a compression test should be given. To do this the patient is lying with his knee on the painful side flexed and his heel on the bed. If the patient's right foot is involved it would be close to the left side of the plinth and you stand at the left side of the patient. You now fixate the cuboid with the right thenar eminence on top and the fingers beneath. The thenar eminence of the other hand together with the fingers grasp the bases and shafts of the 4th and 5th metatarsals. This hand then applies a compression force combined with an antero-posterior glide. (see figure 58)..If pain is produced execute a compression treatment regime as discussed in earlier texts.

(4) The trapezium - 1st metacarpal joint

As all physiotherapists know this is a saddle joint and very prone to degenerative disease. The capsule in the young is slack and it really behaves like a ball and socket joint. If painful the therapist should try a compression test with a view to giving a compression treatment. You hold the seated patient's hand securely to your body. Clasp the trapezium with the

Figure 58

Compression treatment to the cuboid matatarsals joint.

Figure 59

Compression treatment to the trapezium/first metacarpal joint.

thumb and index finger of one hand and the first metacarpal with the thumb and index finger of the other hand (see figure 59). While applying a compressive force, flex and extend then abduct and adduct the thumb to see if it is painful. If so proceed with a compression regime. Provided you follow the 20 second guideline do not be put off by the considerable crepitus sometimes encountered.

(5). The pisiform - triquentrum joint

This joint should not be overlooked when a patient presents with pain in its vicinity. When involved it produces pain with wrist extension especially with passive overpressure as the pisiform is compressed on the carpal beneath. Test this joint by having the patient fully flex the wrist, to relax the structures that stabilise the pisiform, and grasp this small bone with the end pads of the thumb and index finger. It is now compressed on the triquetrum while glided in different directions. If painful apply a compression treatment. I know of no better management.

One interesting case history worth relating was of a lady in her seventies who had complained of pain under the pisiform while in plaster following a Colles fracture. A ridge of the plaster was over the bone in question and the resulting pressure caused the pain which continued after the plaster was removed. Three compression treatments relieved her of all symptoms.

B. PAIN RELEASE PHENOMENON TECHNIQUES - "PRP"s

Apology

Firstly may I apologise for the use of the initials "PRP" but when writing up case notes etc. they are more convenient. Who wants to keep writing Pain Release Phenomenon Techniques out in full all the time. I am sure you will have a place for them after you have read this section and will choose to use the initials.

1. EXPLANATION AND DESCRIPTION

Physiotherapists have been using techniques that are akin to "PRP"s for many years. When frictions are applied to a lesion we all know that if the pressure is constant and not excessive the tenderness experienced will disappear after a short time. In Part 1 of this book I dealt with the acute wry neck and stated that with repeated rotations into the painful range of movement the pain goes. In the section just covered I spoke of the pain release phenomenon we look for within 20 seconds with compression. This latter phenomenon led me to try and see if pain would disappear when provoked in other ways and to my astonishment I found that it did. Because of this exciting find, and the correlation with compression, it had to be covered in this book. As a profession we still have much to learn and do.

At this point in time I would discourage their use as a therapy for acute conditions. They have a place in the treatment of chronic problems when one can assume that the initial stages of repair have taken place. Let me give an example. Say a patient has just torn some fibres in a muscle. An active contraction would be painful as would a passive stretch. Maintaining the contraction or stretch for 20 seconds would not cause a pain release and the chances are that it would make the lesion worse. This is why I use "PRP"s for conditions of longer standing and 6 weeks as a guideline.

Starting with the lower limb and then the upper limb I will give some applications for "PRP"s with a brief case history for interest.

As with other therapies the patient must of course have the purpose of the "PRP"s explained to him. This is because he is expected to feel some discomfort initially and it is important that he informs you as soon as the pain diminishes or goes. When the pain stops it is pointless continuing so they must tell you. You stop and start again. If with your first "PRP" the pain goes in under 6 seconds it may be because you did not provoke enough pain to be useful.

2. SPECIFIC TREATMENT EXAMPLES

(1). Extensor longus hallucis tendinitis

"PRP"s have proved helpful in resolving this condition. The diagnosis is confirmed clinically when resisted active toe extension, palpation and a passive stretch of the tendon are all painful. To treat, you give just enough resistance to active big toe extension to produce a tolerable pain in the tendon. The active contraction is maintained for up to 20 seconds to see if the pain subsides. An explanation is of course given to the patient of what to expect. I usually get more patient involvement by getting them to monitor the time for me with their watch. If the pain disappears the procedure is repeated several times until the movement is virtually painless. It is interesting to note that with each contraction more resistance is required to produce the same level of pain. The next step would be to produce the pain with a stretch. Follow the 20 second rule and if successful repeat several times. At the time of the first visit it may be advisable to use only one procedure. The patients are taught to do their own "PRP"s. This technique would not be used on an acute tendinitis.

(2). Hip pain

Many adults present with hip problems. They may have a capsular pattern loss of movement or have a positive Fabere's sign. "PRP"s can make a dramatic change in the patient's symptoms. The patient would be lying supine. Standing on the unaffected side you flex the hip and knee so that the former is at approximately 90 degrees. A few degrees of adduction is also added. A pad is placed under the patient's buttock on the affected side. One or both of your hands are placed over the flexed knee and a shoulder makes contact with the hand(s) on the knee. (See figure 60). By using the body weight through the hand(s) on the knee a dorsal glide is applied to the hip joint. One is seeking pain with this glide and variations in flexion and/or adduction may be necessary. You apply the "PRP" routine that will now be coming familiar. It is of course of little use in advanced cases of arthritis and what is more you would not receive a favourable response within the 20 seconds.

The next procedure would be for a patient with a positive Fabere's test. Place him in this test position and then press his knee towards the plinth

Figure 60

"PRP" hip joint. Postero-lateral glide of femur.

Figure 61

"PRP" to hip joint in Fabere position.

seeking pain at a tolerable level. (See figure 61). Maintaining it for the "magical" 20 seconds see if it responds favourably. If so proceed and the knee will move closer to the plinth and the patient will arise feeling much better. You sometimes get fabulous results. Another way to "PRP" is, when in the Fabere position, have the patient actively abduct against resistance that you apply. If this produces pain have him hold the contraction for up to 20 seconds and see if the pain subsides. It usually will and subsequent contractions bring the knee closer to the bed. "PRP"s offer much to the therapist and patient in the management of hip pain.

(3). De Quervain's disease (stenosing tenovaginitis)

This painful condition is difficult to treat and often requires surgical intervention. However I would suggest you include in your therapy "PRP"s. To do this have the patient make a fist with the thumb inside the fingers. You now deviate the wrist medially until a tolerable level of pain is produced. The patient can in fact do this with the other hand. The "PRP"s are now under way.

(4). Tennis Elbow

With all "PRP"s, as the reader will now be aware, the contractions or stretches which reproduce the pain are sought and from these the treatment strategy is planned. For "tennis elbow" I would suggest that you make use of the tests used in making the diagnosis.

Many patients experience pain with resisted extension of the 4th and/or 3rd fingers. This discomfort is usually worse in full extension of the elbow but you would start at 90 degrees, if this was also pain positive, and use "PRP"s on the painful responses using one finger at a time. The patient is taught to do them and instructed to repeat the program six times a day. Patients responding to this program report pleasing daily progress and it becomes necessary for them to extend the arm further to reproduce the pain. Use is made of other pain provoking movements such as wrist extension with a clenched fist.

However the reader will recall that earlier in this book a new approach in the treatment of tennis elbow was using mobilisations with movement. MWMs should be tried first and if unsuccessful then try the above.

(5). Golfer's Elbow

I first used "PRP"s on a 40 years old patient who, as the result of a direct blow to the medial aspect of his elbow was suffering from a medial epicondylitis. This condition had bothered him for over four months and failed to respond to medication. On examination he was unable to flex his fingers or wrist against any resistance without considerable pain. On the day of his first visit he had ultrasound and then "PRP"s for wrist and finger flexion. He was an intelligent patient and was both interested and pleased with his response to this new therapy. He quickly learned to "PRP" himself. Two days later he was virtually pain free and no further treatments were given. This proved to me beyond reasonable doubt that "PRP"s were a valuable adjunct to our therapies.

(6). The chronic painful shoulder

This is indeed a vague heading but I have had some super results using "PRP"s on many of the different conditions that befall the shoulder joint. I seek the static contractions or stretch movements that produce pain and look for the 20 seconds or less response. One procedure that I have found of great value has been to have the patient supine on the plinth with his elbow fully flexed and the shoulder flexed to 90 degrees. I am referring to the painful side of course. You stand at the good side and place one hand over the patient's elbow and the other under his scapular. (See figure 62). Use your body weight to glide the humeral head posteriorly seeking pain. It may be necessary to add some horizontal flexion to the humerus to provoke discomfort. When painful sustain for up to 20 seconds to see if the desired pain disappearance occurs. The procedure is similar to that used on the hip and described earlier. This has proved very useful with some chronic rotator cuff lesions.

Figure 62

A "PRP" for the shoulder joint. Similar to hip technique.

3. CONCLUSION

The most exciting thing about "PRP"s is that like other forms of manual therapy the therapist can expect some change at the time of delivery when they are indicated. I laboured this point when dealing with "NAGS" and "SNAGS". However they should not be used to the exclusion of other physical therapies.

The biggest problem that therapists will have with "PRP"s will be judging the amount of resistance to give when applying them or how much stretch to use. It is better to start with too little than too much. If too little the pain produced may only take a few seconds to disappear. One would of course, if this were the case, apply stronger resistance or a stronger stretch the next time. Too much sustained resistance could exacerbate the lesion and "PRP"s might have to be discarded.

I did say at the beginning that "PRP"s were still in the development stage. This "magical" time of 20 seconds may need reconsidering. There have been times with very chronic conditions when I have lingered longer with good results but there will always be exceptions to rules. I have also mentioned that in the early stages of soft tissue injuries they should not be used but maybe if done gently and looking for say a 5 second pain relief response they may have a place in speeding up recovery. I would hesitate to try them within 48 hours of injury bearing in mind the R.I.C.E. advice. At this point in time my most spectacular results have been with conditions of many months standing.

C. OTHER EXTREMITY THERAPIES

Explanation

In this final section I wish to refer to assorted techniques that the reader will find of interest. This will further explain the use of the term pot pourri in the heading of Part 2. Not to be missed is the "SQUEEZE" technique for the knee and the strappings for heel pain and achilles tendinitis.

1. PLANTAR FASCIITIS - HEEL PAIN

In the November 1973 issue of the N.Z. Journal of Physiotherapy I had published an article titled " 'Plantar Fasciitis': A Study Report". (8) This article dealt with heel pain and the inference was that most patients diagnosed as having plantar fasciitis did not in fact have this condition but instead a joint problem. The sub talar joints were involved and causing the pain and not the plantar fascia. I drew this conclusion from the fact that most patients presenting with heel pain responded to manual therapy to these joints together with exercises and footwear advice.

Figure 63
Taping for heel pain.

Years later nothing has happened to make me change my mind and in this respect I have the support of many colleagues.

In this edition I wish to add the strapping that I use for heel pain. It can be so effective that when applied, patients who have limped into my rooms have walked out with no pain. The tape is used to alter the position of the calcaneum in relation to the talus. This is achieved by taping the calcaneum in external rotation. Two strips (approximately 2 cms wide) are used. The first is placed obliquely around the back of the heel, and while the calcaneum is forcibly externally rotated, the tape is wrapped up around the lower leg to maintain the position. The second tape is applied over the first to make the fixation even more effective. (See figure 63) When the patients stand they initially have difficulty walking because of the re-positioning but no pain should be felt. The tape is left for 48 hour and the result noted. It is part of the treatment routine for heel pain and may have to be used for a week or two.

2. THE "SQUEEZE" TECHNIQUE FOR THE KNEE

Introduction

The origin of this treatment must be told and before doing so I would again remind the reader of that famous quote attributed to Louis Pasteur : " In the field of discovery chance only favours the prepared mind". About four years ago we were treating a grubby 25 year old male with a knee joint "derangement". He twisted it playing football resulting in loss of at least 25 degrees of extension and 35 degrees of flexion. Some hours after his injury the knee became swollen and he had a noticeable bulge over the antero - medial joint margin. An appointment had been made for him to see an Orthopaedic surgeon and pending this visit he was referred to us for therapy. Our management included the usual manual techniques one may try to restore knee movement, ultrasound and of course quadriceps and hamstring exercises. The therapy was useless and resulted in the patient understandably complaining after five visits that he would be wasting his time by attending further. We readily agreed with him and asked him to maintain an exercise program at home until assessed by the surgeon. As a final gesture I decided to again check his knee. I used the McMurray test and applied a very firm pressure over the anterior horn where the prominent bulge was located. To my amazement his knee flexed fully, without pain, and what was even more amazing I was able to then extend it fully from the flexed position. It must be added that I did not release my firm thumb pressure over the anterior horn. The patient was understandably delighted. "I'm cured!" he exclaimed. "Of course!" was my nonchalant reply. It was then pointed out to this fellow that only a temporary resolution to his problem had been brought about and he could expect further trouble if he twisted his knee again. He demanded after this "miracle" a return appointment two days later which was agreed to. He was fine and required neither further therapy nor surgery and I must add that he did not appear to be so grubby?

Referring again to my quotation above may I say that I most certainly had a prepared mind. From that time the "Squeeze" technique has been an important and rewarding part of my therapy for knees that have lost flexion and in many cases can be helpful in restoring extension.

The "Squeeze" for flexion can be applied in lying or standing but for extension is only done in lying.

Knee flexion is tested in lying and partial weightbearing for a movement loss or pain. When we ask the standing patient to squat down we have them hold on to any secure object(s) at the same time so they are only partially weight bearing. Full weight bearing may not only be too painful but there is a risk of exacerbating the condition. If the restriction and pain is present when lying then your treatment is done in this position. If the loss and pain is only evident when weightbearing then the "Squeeze" would be applied with the patient standing. Please be mindful of the contraindications to manual therapy and if you have any doubts always give a trial treatment with the patient supine. The treatment is always uncomfortable but should be well tolerated by the patient.

Before describing the procedure I would draw your attention to the fact that when a knee is put through a full range of movement there is always a position through this range when you can palpably feel some joint space between the femur and tibia. This is because of the very convex shape of the femoral facet and the way the joint behaves biomechanically. In full flexion for instance it is easy to palpate the joint space over the anterior horn of the meniscus (medial or lateral), but with extension this cannot be done as the tibia and femur approximate. One makes use of this knowledge, as the "Squeeze" is applied when you feel there is space available beneath the fingertips during the range of movement.

Description for a loss of flexion

The supine patient's knee is palpated around the medial and lateral joint margins seeking an area of local tenderness. If located over the postero - medial joint space of the right knee you stand at the left side of the pa-

Figure 64

"Squeeze" technique for the knee. Medial "derangement" in lying.

tient. Place the terminal pad of one thumb, reinforced by the other, over the joint margin where it is tender. The patient now actively flexes his knee and when you feel the joint space open up beneath your thumbs you squeeze centrally. At the same time you encourage additional joint flexion with the ulnar border of your hand that is lying over the upper end of the tibia. (See figure 64). Maintain the squeeze and overpressure for a few seconds and repeat three times before reassessing the range of movement. Patients will always feel discomfort which is understandable but it is a tolerable procedure and if not you would not use it. If the pain and palpable tenderness was over the lateral joint margin you would stand on the same side to enable you to use your thumbs to apply the squeeze. The thumbs are used because they are stronger than the fingers.

If the pain and/or loss of movement is when weightbearing only then the "Squeeze" is done while the patient squats down. Kneel at your patient's feet (help from above?) and place your thumbs over the joint margin where you suspect attention is needed. As the patient squats you apply thumb pressure as the joint space becomes available. (See figure 65). Remember to have the patient holding on to something to avoid full weight bearing. This weightbearing variation would also be used as a progression on the supine position if you thought it necessary. Words like exciting should not be used in a textbook to describe what so often hap-

Figure 65

"Squeeze" technique in partial weightbearing for medial joint signs.

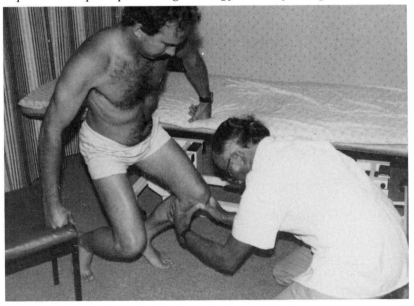

pens with this technique. However when you can markedly increase the flexion in a knee with a "Squeeze" that has been absent for 8 years and do this in the presence of many colleagues why not? May I again remind the reader that if the squeeze discomfort increases as a patient bends his knee abandon the technique as you must with other therapies covered in this book. If there is no improvement in range at the time of delivery then try something else. An alternative way to "Squeeze" in weightbearing is to have the patient place her foot on the affected side on a chair. She can hold on to the back of the chair when leaning forward over her knee while you "Squeeze".

Explanation

I am always asked when teaching what I think this technique is doing when one considers the known pathologies that occur within the knee. The menisci as we know are wedge shaped. Perhaps a new type of mechanical lesion called "a meniscal segment displacement" should be considered. Perhaps with a weightbearing twist of the knee a segment of a meniscus can when squeezed displace minimally in a peripheral direction. It could even do this sometimes when the meniscus is torn. This would explain why squeezing in a remedial direction can spectacularly correct this anomaly if it exists. It works, perhaps you have a better explanation?

3. THE STIFF SHOULDER

In the mid 1970's I wrote an article for The NZ Journal of Physiotherapy (10) on the use of a stick to encourage external rotation in the shoulder joint. All physiotherapists know that a loss of this movement is always seen in capsular lesions and may in fact be the only movement restriction in patients with shoulder pathology. Also known is the need for external rotation when the arm is elevated through abduction.

I am including this exercise because in my mind the Pain Release Phenomenon is encountered in yet another form. (cf. Acute Wry Neck).

The patient is supine on a plinth with his shoulder abducted to 90 degrees and the elbow over the edge. A stick is placed upright on the floor. The base of it is out from the shoulder and stabilised with some sandbags. A broom or mop could just as easily be used. The other end is clasped by the patient with the elbow at a right angle. (See figure 66). The patient now carries out external rotation exercises for up to 20 minutes. It helps if some heat can be applied at the same time. The repetitions when done diligently always result in an increase in external rotation provided no increase in pain with exercise is experienced due perhaps to over enthusiasm. As the minutes tick by, most patients are pleased as they feel less

Figure 66

Stick exercises for external rotation of the shoulder joint.

movement discomfort ("PRP"?) and note an increased range. It is great as a home exercise when a broom or mop is used on a carpeted floor. Monitor the patients as they tend to extend the elbow which converts the motion into abduction. However if abduction were required as might be the case after immobilisation following a dislocated shoulder then the exercise can be done with the elbow extended. In this case the pole should be held with the arm well short of external rotation.

Note! If the base of the pole is moved towards the foot of the bed then gravity would assist the movement. If it is shifted towards the head of the bed more muscle effort is required.

4. THE ACROMIO - CLAVICULAR JOINT

According to some anatomists this joint can have a meniscus and I would agree. Often after trauma it responds to a technique I evolved to mobilise the joint and deal with it if deranged. The procedure takes into account the fact that when the arm is fully elevated the clavicle externally rotates. If this rotation is blocked and the arm elevated actively with some momentum, at the end of the motion an additional rotation will take place at the acromio-clavicular joint. It is the momentum that makes this happen. If you try this on a normal joint you can invariably produce a crepitus. With the injured joint it tends to remain silent if it is hypomobile but after a few swings with clavicular fixation it frees and the patient is instantly much better.

To do this have the patient seated. Stand behind him and to one side and fixate the clavicle on the other side with the ulnar border of your hand. (See figure 67). The patient now swings his arm up in front of him towards full elevation. He must not be too vigorous. It is important that the therapist does not stand behind the arm being elevated for fear of being struck in the face. However one blow will ensure compliance. I usually have them swing a few times seeking the return of the crepitus. If the patient found it too painful then follow the golden rule and desist.

Figure 67

Fixation for patient mobilisation of the acromio-clavicular joint.

EPILOGUE

This book was written with one purpose in mind and that was to acquaint the reader with the techniques of the author. Many of these have not been published and those that have been are difficult to assemble. The contents could have included copious details of pertinent anatomy and biomechanics but this background material is well known to physiotherapists and there are always many excellent texts available.

My most valuable self learning and teaching tools are my articulated plastic spine and the articulated bones of the upper and lower extremity. Being flexible and accurate in detail makes it simple for me to show and explain to patients what I propose to do. This is especially true for "NAGS", "SNAGS" and "MWM"s.

After presenting a paper on "SNAGS" (11) at the 1988 IFOMT World Congress in Cambridge, England I was asked by many participants what the initials NAG stood for. There is of course a tale related to this. For years when recording manual techniques I have related many of them to the source. A Kaltenborn technique was often prefixed with the initials Kb, a Maitland technique would be prefixed with Mait or a McConnell with McC. With my original neck mobilisations I cheekily thought of calling them Nagillums which of course is Mulligan spelt backwards. My colleague of the day, Trish Gardiner, said the word was far too long and shortened it to NAGS. Some years later a bright colleague suggested that NAG could be an acronym for the words Natural Apophyseal Glides which says it all.

Much of what is covered in this book will eventually be supported following sound clinical trials and I look forward to the future with confidence and enthusiasm. There is still so much to discover and learn.

REFERENCES

(1) Kaltenborn F M, Mobilisation of the Extremity Joints. Oslo: Olaf Norlis Bokhandel, 1980

(2) McKenzie R A, The Lumbar Spine: Waikanae, Spinal Publications, 1981

(3) Mulligan B R, The Acute Wry Neck: New Zealand Journal of Physiotherapy, May, 1957

(4) Mooney V, Where is the Pain Coming From?: Spine 12;8,1987

(5) Grieve G P, Modern Manual Therapy: Edinburgh, Churchill Livingstone, 1986

(6) Maitland G D, The Hypothesis of Adding Compression When Examining and Treating Synovial Joints: The Journal of Orthopaedic and Sports Physical Therapy: 2.1.1980

(7) McConnell J, The Management of Chondromalacia Patellae-A Long Term Solution: Published proceedings of MTAA biennial conference Brisbane1985

(8) Mulligan B R, Plantar Fasciitis?: A Study Report: New Zealand Journal of Physiotherapy, November, 1973

(9) Mennell J McM, Joint Pain: Boston, Little Brown,1964

(10) Mulligan B R, The Painful Stiff Shoulder: New Zealand Journal of Physiotherapy, 4.7.1974

(11) Mulligan B R, "SNAGS", Published papers IFOMT Congress, 1988